Vixen
Unleashed

Find Your Inner Sexy. Lose Your Outer Fat.
The 12-Week Weight Loss Road Trip To Freedom!

By

Lynne Sadowski

with Keesha Ewers, PhD., ANRP

Please seek advice from a medical doctor prior to starting any weight loss program or making dietary changes. The opinions in this book are not intended as a substitute for professional dietary counseling or medical services. The author has made every effort to ensure validity, accuracy, and safety of the information presented here. However, no guarantee is made that the techniques described are suitable for everybody, or that specific results will be achieved. The authors and publishers of this book shall be held harmless and without fault in all situations arising from the use of this information by any given person with or without medical supervision.

Illustrations by Rae Edwards

Cover Art by Roxanne Gordon and Courtney Sotack – Cover Photography by Todd Sadowski

Copyright © 2012 Lynne Sadowski

All rights reserved.

ISBN: 1480228206

ISBN 13:   9781480228207

Dedication

This book is dedicated to my son, Jake. Dream big.
Believe in yourself. Live your life with passion.
Never give up.
Trust your instinct. Know that you will always be okay.
And never forget that *my* biggest dream is to give *you* the
world! I love you more than life, itself. - *Mom*

Contents

INTRODUCTION
MAPPING OUT THE ROAD TRIP

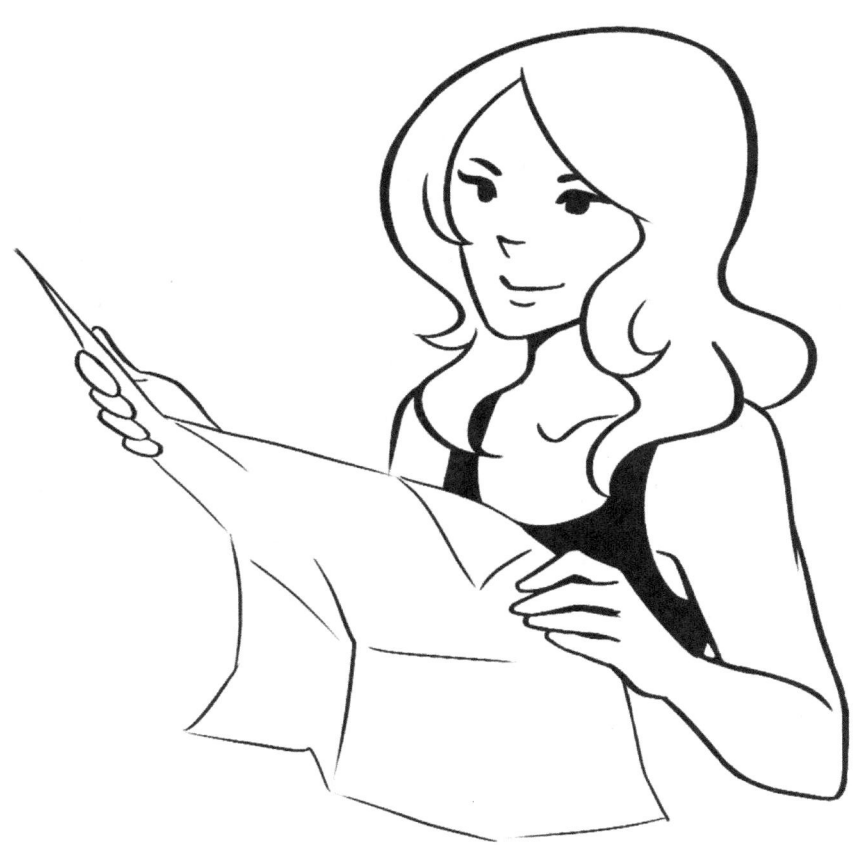

What woman hasn't had days, or even weeks when she's wanted to run away from it all...Like the girl in a relationship that's gone stale, and daydreams about meeting a gorgeous new man who comes in and sweeps her off her feet. Or the woman who works 50+ hours per week and hates her job; she fantasizes about the day she tells her *real* feelings to the boss, and clocks out for the last time. And then there's the woman who has just too much on her plate. She's ready to say, "P%#K it", drive off into the sunset, and never look back. Do any of these women sound like you?

When your life is out of whack or in constant chaos, your immune system breaks down, you get sick, and you get fat. If you're suffering from chronic health issues, or you've had a lifetime of yo-yo dieting, there is a good chance that something a little deeper is going on. You see, to put it simply, your outer state (your body) is a complete reflection of your inner state. So, if you want to change your body and your health, and get rid of the chaos in your life, you'll first need to reconnect with that incredible woman who lies deep in your soul, and do some serious healing. It's time for you to find your true, feminine self and create a life and body that reflect your ***real*** spirit.

Before you read another page of *Vixen Unleashed*, you need to know that we won't be tackling weight loss in your typical fashion, with ***just*** diet and exercise. That is only a part of the process. This will be a journey of the mind, the body, and the spirit. So I ask that you go into this with an open mind. In addition to helping you achieve a stronger, healthier, and thinner body, I am going to be sharing valuable information to help you grow stronger mentally, emotionally and spiritually, as well.

When working on improving their health, many women will ignore the "spirit" part of the catch phrase, "Mind, Body, Spirit". Most are willing to workout and eat healthy for the welfare of their bodies, and some are willing to instill positive attitudes for the welfare of their minds. However, all three elements of this trio are important to you becoming a whole and healthy woman. No matter what you call it... God, the Universe, or The Man Upstairs... Something greater than us *does* exist. There is an energy force that surrounds us, and flows within us. This *presence* resides in each of us individually, yet unites us all, collectively. What you may not know is that there are two sides to our Higher Power: the Divine Feminine and the Divine Masculine. Also known in some cultures as the Yin/Yang, when these two aspects of the Universe are not in balance, we experience stress in our bodies, our lives, and our planet. For thousands of years, the Divine Masculine has been our dominating Source. However, it is believed that the Mayan calendar ending on December 21, 20*12*, was not an indication of the end of our world, but rather, the beginning of a universal shift, and a resurgence of the Divine Feminine into our lives!

Over the centuries, our global culture has been heavily ruled with masculine influence: competition, wars, achievement, linear business models, structured work, and muscular bodies. While our nurturing, we-centered, organic, and intuitive nature has been suppressed. Both Universal polarities, when working synergistically, offer Divine grace; but when the scale is constantly tipped in either one or the other direction, that's when you find chaos.

More and more, we are seeing a change in gender roles. We women are not only working and earning a living; we are becoming household breadwinners and leaders in business and politics! However, while we've been advancing swiftly, enjoying all of the opportunities that previously were only given to men, our feminine principles have been greatly stifled, creating an imbalance that actually inhibits us from reaching our true potential and seeing even greater successes in life. So, YES!! Become astronauts and engineers. Climb mountains and win Presidencies! But don't lose sight of who we are at our core...don't lose sight of our natural, God-given blessings as women. When we bring our feminine energies into our masculine, achievement-driven world...that's when we unleash our true power, and begin to see the changes that we desire.

Desiring change is not a bad thing at all. And it's perfectly okay to want a healthier, leaner body. However, what is *not* okay, is expecting our bodies to be something they are *not* meant to be. Not every woman is destined to have abs of steel. Not every woman is born to have long, muscular legs. Some are, and some aren't. One of my visions in *Vixen Unleashed* is to help you realize your true self… *whatever that may be*. Whether you're curvy and soft, or super lean and athletic, you are who you are. And we are all different. As your coach on this journey, I hope to help you live to be authentically YOU… and a healthier, stronger, sexier, and leaner version of YOU, as well. I aim to help you find that Divine Feminine inside and bring "sexy" back into your life.

Being sexy is not about fitting into your skinny jeans. True sexiness is not a physical state at all; rather, it is a *state of being*. It goes way beyond body size. Being a *Vixen* is exerting that state of being; it's expressing an aura of confidence, inner beauty, and knowingness. A Vixen has a charisma and an energy about her that's indescribable. How do you connect with *your* feminine energy to become a Vixen? It begins with looking within, and uncovering truth. And to be a *Vixen Unleashed,* is to know who you are, own it, and then live it. *Vixen Unleashed* is a truly a way of life. And to truly take hold of this lifestyle, you must practice what I call, "sensual living".

What is sensual living? Think about it this way: When you are having the most incredible, loving sex, you embrace all of your senses in that moment. Your mind isn't racing - you're not thinking about work, the kids, or the errands you need to run. You let yourself go, and you *feel* the heat between the two of you, as the temperature rises. You *smell* his hair, his cologne, and his masculine scent. You *hear* his heart pounding, and *taste* his salty skin as you kiss his neck. You *look* at his muscles ripple as he moves, and you *see* his soul through his eyes. And when you engage in your "sixth" sense, you become *connected spiritually* as well. This is sexy; THIS is **sensual**! However, embracing life like this is not limited to sexual interludes only. Imagine how extraordinary life would be if you could experience sensual living in everything you do!

⌒⌒

— Sensual living is SEXY living. It's slowing down and embracing life and all its beauty, igniting your senses and being keenly aware, in every moment. —

⌒⌒

WHAT TO EXPECT

Welcome to *Vixen Unleashed…Find your inner sexy. Lose your outer fat.* Get ready to go on a 12-week weight loss road trip that begins in your Comfort Zone and ends in the town of Freedom. As you travel throughout this journey, you'll gain insight on how to live life more sensually. If you are ready to find freedom from what is really causing you to be fat, you must be willing to look inside and become honest with yourself, and then do the work. This is a more than just a weight-loss journey. It's a road trip… complete with detours, mile markers, maps, roadblocks, and a super hot convertible with a V*12* engine! Together, we're going down Interstate Vixen12 where you will unleash your inner Vixen and experience *sexy* in a whole new way!

If you had asked me several years ago, I would never have considered myself sexy. Although I had a great job and family, and seemed to be living a dream life, I was overweight and miserable and felt extremely unattractive. As a result of working long hours and burning the candle at both ends, I had grown physically and emotionally stressed and unhealthy. I had consistently put everyone and everything ahead of myself and it finally caught up with me. Then a series of events occurred that led to the moment, which turned my life around. That was the day I unleashed my inner Vixen.

If you've never known your inner Vixen, or perhaps it's just been a while since you've seen her, things are about to change. If you are anything like I was, you may be wondering why your health has taken a back seat in life. It's simple - we women have been conditioned throughout our lives to be super heroes. We work full time jobs, raise children, join all the committees, run to soccer games and dance recitals, take care of all the errands and household chores. On top of that, we bust our butts to prove ourselves in the workplace by taking on more responsibilities, and working harder. And what woman doesn't pride herself on her ability to multi-task? It is so ingrained in our lifestyle and culture that we even list "great multi-tasker" on our resumes! But too often the reason we are performing all of these tasks is to please somebody other than ourselves. We repeatedly set aside our own needs to take care of everyone else. Then, when we can't fit everything into a day, we get frustrated and beat ourselves up for not being able to do it all. We are stressed by the demands of the world and find it impossible to say, "no". But the truth is, the mental and emotional stress we endure is primarily caused by our own choices in life. We *choose* to work harder, *choose* to over-schedule, and *choose* to eat fast food for convenience. In case you haven't heard, stress causes fat; especially that fat that surrounds our mid-section and puts us at risk of heart disease and premature death. So if we are *choosing* to create stress in our lives, we are essentially *choosing* to be fat. I'm not placing blame on you AT ALL for being fat. There is no blame...it just *is*. I'm saying that once we recognize that everything we do in life is a choice, then we can consciously begin making new choices. And after years of making the wrong choices, this transition will not be easy. We have consistently made the decision to put our health and well being last on the priority list. And it's time for change. However, to get out of this situation, you're going to have to leave your comfort zone, take yourself out of the back seat, and put yourself into the driver's seat!

Vixen Unleashed is an exciting road trip! Soon you'll discover that your waistline isn't the cause of your stress, but the *result*. In these pages, you'll be getting tools that you need to shift your paradigms once and for all. You will learn more about who you are and understand how you got here today. There are many diet and exercise programs out there that work… if you stick to them. But, the real reason so many women cannot stick with a long-term plan is because many of these weight-loss programs don't teach you to go inward, make adjustments in your mindset, and connect with your inner spirit. This is more than just a diet. It's a journey of life transformation. I've created a plan that is as balanced as I strive for your life to be.

So, to ensure you are getting everything you need to be successful in this program, I'm giving you a **diet** to follow, an **exercise plan** to implement, **strategies** to help **change your thinking**, and tools to help you **reconnect with your Inner Vixen**! Mind. Body. Spirit…all in balance! Your 12-week program will encompass both masculine and feminine qualities. There will be structure and goal setting (masculine). There will also be introspection and flexibility (feminine). During each week of the *Vixen Unleashed* program, you will learn new tricks and tools to re-shape your life, like how to be grateful for the life that brought you to this point. You will develop a vision for who you want to be, and use that vision to spur you on in making choices that drive you straight to your goal. You will shift your gears and reverse your conditioning. You will learn to take ownership of where you are now, and realize the only person who can change your direction forever is YOU. Whether you overeat as a way to cope, you hate to exercise, or you've always put yourself last on the list, you will develop the skills to overcome these issues. If you've struggled all your life with the burden of excess weight, this can be the start of a personal revolution! In the following pages we will be taking a good old-fashioned road trip, and along the way you will uncover the tools you need to lose excess body fat. But don't think that's all you're going to lose! You'll also be shedding the *F*ears, *A*ttitudes, and *T*oxic behaviors that brought you here in the first place. At the end of each week in the road trip, you will encounter a Mile Marker. This is where you'll find your action steps that are designed to give you more confidence, change the way you think, and help you create the body you desire and life you deserve. So, if you've ever wanted to run away from it all, now is the time. Get ready for a road trip. Get ready to become a *Vixen Unleashed*!

Chapter 1

The Day I Unleashed My Inner Vixen

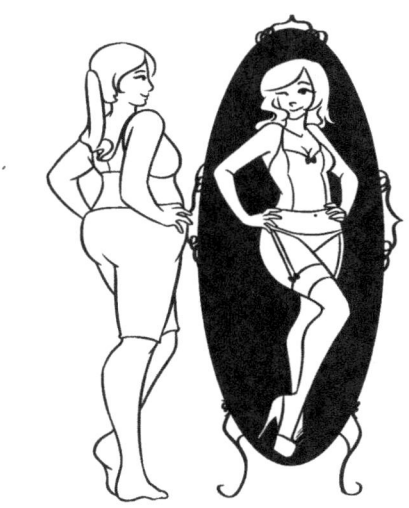

aised in a small town in North Carolina, as a young girl I fantasized that I would grow up to be beautiful, smart and confident. I lived for opportunities to dance and perform "shows" for my family in the living room. Being front and center stage was where I was born to be. Like many little girls, I fantasized about being someone really awesome when I got older. Only instead of Barbie, or a princess, I imagined myself to be a famous stage actress, or a soap star like the ones Mom and I would watch on daytime TV. My inspiration at the time was Hope Brady, a character on *Days of our Lives*. She was intelligent, beautiful, and sexy; but best of all; she was married to super-hot, ex biker-boy turned cop, Bo Brady. (Maybe he's the reason that I went for those biker guy types in my early twenties)

From the time I was four years old, I knew I wanted to one day leave my small town for a life in the entertainment industry. By the time I turned eleven, I started taking acting classes at a community theater about 40 minutes from my house. Knowing how much I wanted to be an actress, Mom ensured that I never missed one acting class, audition, or rehearsal. Since the theater was so far from home, whenever I had a class or rehearsal, Mom would just sit in the car and read a book while she waited for me to finish up. Then, at sunset we would trek another 40 minutes back home. I didn't realize until later in life (and until becoming a mom, myself) what kind of love she must have had for me, to go out of her way like that, day after day and week after week. She always called me a dreamer. And, gratefully, neither of my parents ever discouraged me from following my dreams. I think that's why, throughout my life, I have always encouraged all the people around me to do the same. Even back then, I held a strong belief that a person could do anything they wanted in life, as long as they had a vision, belief in themselves, and determination. Mom and Dad supported my dream as I continued performing throughout my Junior High and High School years.

After High School I moved to New York to attend acting school. That's when my weight struggles all began. Up until then, I had always been quite skinny, but like any teen going away to college, I learned to eat cheaply; and in New York City, affordable, accessible foods such as pizza and bagels created the perfect recipe for me to put on the "freshman 15". (Although for me, it turned out to be more like the "freshman 50"!) Moving away to a big city like New York was intimidating for an 18-year old small-town girl, and the pressures of school and living in the Big Apple were a challenge for me. I think it was the first time in my life that I really experienced significant stress. So, not only was I eating certain foods because they were cheap, I was eating them for emotional reasons too. I just didn't realize it. Being overweight was something I had never dealt with before. I didn't understand anything about healthy portions or unhealthy food choices. I ate what I wanted, when I wanted, and how much I wanted. As the months rolled by during the school year, the stress intensified, and my clothes got tighter, until the time came that I could barely squeeze into anything anymore. The more the pressures increased, the more my appetite did. As I couldn't afford to buy new clothes, my wardrobe staple became an old pair of baggy overalls that I borrowed from my roommate. Those overalls hid everything. They concealed my fat well, but they also hid the truth: I was struggling in school and couldn't handle big city life.

Given my budget, my living situation was less than glamorous. When I first moved to New York, my parents helped me settle into a room that I rented at the YMCA on 34th street. I made a few close friends there, who also attended my school. The rooms were tiny, and there were showers and bathroom stalls on every floor that we shared with other girls. After a while, my new friends and I were tired of the cramped living and decided to move into an apartment together; so we set out to find something that we all could afford. We finally settled on an apartment just outside of Spanish Harlem. It wasn't the best place to live, for three naive kids who were new to New York. But we liked it…for a while. Soon after we moved, however a series of events occurred that brought me close to my emotional limits: both of my roommates were mugged at gunpoint in my neighborhood, and then our heating system broke during the middle of a cold, New York winter. We were freezing, but no matter how much we complained, our landlord wouldn't do anything about it. And on top of that, our apartment was infested with mice! The last straw for me was the night I saw a mouse scamper across my bed. It was then that I decided to finally call it quits; I just pulled the covers over my head and sobbed. I couldn't take it any more.

I didn't want to give up my dreams of being an entertainer, but living in New York was not for me. Sometimes you have to make choices as to what is more important to you in life. I'm happy that I made the decision to leave school, and I never regretted it. I dropped out of school and bought a one-way bus ticket home to North Carolina. I had to give the overalls back to my girlfriend, and the only article of clothing I owned that fit me anymore was my bathrobe. So I packed my bags, put on my robe, boarded the Greyhound and headed back home. I was pathetic. It was a long ride home that night and I did a lot of thinking. I knew that leaving school was the right thing for me, but I felt like I had let down my family and friends. I was far from the starlet that I had set out to be when I left my small town.

Not long after arriving back into North Carolina, I read about a casting call for a film that was shooting in a nearby town for a woman my age. I wanted to audition but was hesitant because of my weight. Eventually, I mustered up the courage, and went for a try-out. I did well, and after a few rounds, the casting director had narrowed the selections down to another girl and myself. I remember after the final read-through, the casting director pulled me aside and told me that I was clearly a better actress, but that they were looking for someone thinner. They gave the part to the other woman. That pain of being rejected *because* of my weight was a very strong motivator to lose it. It was after that audition that I spent 3 months at home, rarely leaving the house. I stayed in my parents' house and dedicated my time to exercise and diet until I lost the weight. At 19 years old and living back with Mom and Dad, it was not too difficult to shed the pounds. It's a lot easier to accomplish weight loss goals when you don't have a job, a mortgage, a family, and responsibilities.

During those three months I had it good. My mom was my personal chef and the half hour exercise show on TV at 7 AM and 7 PM was my personal trainer. I was very lucky, and my mom was so great to me. I remember once, she drove three hours down to the Stouffer's outlet in South Carolina just to buy me a freezer full of frozen low calorie meals for my lunches. Every day she made me healthy dinners with fruit and fresh salads. She felt my pain and wanted to help. In no time at all, my weight was back to normal and my life as a fat girl was over… or so I thought.

Instead, that is when the roller coaster of weight gain and loss really began. Although I had lost a lot of weight, eventually it came back. Looking back, the big problem wasn't even the fat itself; it was my self-esteem. Going away to college and failing to accomplish what I had set out to do in life was a huge disappointment. Not only had I dropped out of acting school, I buried my feelings in food. Like many women, I became an emotional eater. I ate to cope with my feelings. I started believing that I was destined to always be a fat girl. From then on, my weight would yo-yo. Eventually, even during times when I was thin, I didn't believe that I was attractive and I still saw that "fat girl" every time I looked in the mirror. My confidence was gone.

In my early twenties I was involved in an unhealthy relationship that became the catalyst for a change that ushered in one of the happiest times in my life. I lived with a man who was manipulative and controlling, and he knew I wasn't happy with him. He constantly made "fat" comments, whether or not I was heavy. What I came to realize was that his words were intended to keep me under his control. If I felt that I was unworthy of a decent relationship (because of my appearance) then in his mind, I wouldn't leave him. So, he made verbal digs every chance he could. However, somewhere…somehow… I finally worked up the courage to leave him, and I began by searching for my own place to live. As I scoured the classifieds for an apartment, I stumbled upon a job posting seeking flight attendants. "Wow! What a great idea… I could get out of an "F"-d up relationship AND get paid for it!", I thought. So I applied, interviewed, and got the job. It didn't matter that I had a fear of flying; at that point I would have done anything to get away from this guy! It was one of the best moves I ever made in my life.

For the first time in a long time, I had a sense of freedom. I didn't turn to food for comfort because I was really happy with my accomplishments and myself. Eating food became a way to sustain my energy and I spent that energy enjoying life, and focusing on meeting new people and seeing new places. Food preparation was part of my ritual, just like brushing my teeth. I could have easily used the excuse that I didn't have time to eat right because I travel, but I prepared and packed food and chose my trips based on layovers where I could eat healthy and get some sort of exercise. Exercise wasn't always working out in a gym, either. Sometimes it was running outside or on my treadmill, with my trusty Walkman in hand. And most of the time, I worked up my sweat going to *Hammerjack's*, the local nightclub in Baltimore (where I lived at the time), dancing the night away!

I didn't dread exercise or feel deprived. I didn't eat right just to stay thin, nor did I feel guilty if I had a candy bar. I made healthy eating choices 90% of the time simply because it felt right and it felt good. After a while, it became second nature. I ate healthy and exercised because that was a way to take care of someone I loved - *myself*. I can honestly say that during this time in my life I felt like the woman I always wanted to be. I loved my body and enjoyed just being alive. I was at the top of my game. Life was good. I was healthy and happy, thin, confident and sexy. I was the person I imagined myself to be. I guess you could say that I was a Vixen!

The dramatic change I went through made me realize that when you have self-confidence, it radiates through your attitude, your outward appearance, and in your body language. Soon I discovered that it also brings dating to a whole new level! I realized that I could be as picky as I wanted to be. I did not have to settle for just anyone! I went out with several different guys during my flight attendant years. After my previous relationship, I didn't really have the desire to get serious with anyone right away. I wasn't looking for my prince charming. I simply enjoyed just being single for a while; I went out with a pilot, a doctor, and other professionals - I went out with bartenders and musicians too. There was even a 5-month stint when I dated a lead guitar player from one of the hottest rock bands in the mid '80's! That was pretty cool, because when I wasn't traveling for my job, I was seeing the countryside by tour-bus. But that all changed the day I met Brett. He was one of the most incredible people I had ever met. He always had a smile on his face and looked at the goodness in everything and everybody. He was a musician too...but at a local level, so he didn't make much money. However, I would always encourage him to pursue his music career. It was his passion. I have wonderful memories of our time together, but there was one time in particular that I'll never forget. He showed up at my apartment one day, out of the blue with a dozen yellow roses (my favorite!!). There was no particular reason for the flowers, so I asked why he bought them for me. I told him he shouldn't be spending his money on flowers and reminded him that he wasn't rich! I'll never forget his answer, "As long as I have you in my life, I'll always be rich." I know what you're thinking... what a line! Although Brett *was* being his silly-self with that comment, he meant every word of it. That was just the way he was...it's interesting that after many years of meeting Mr. Wrong, it wasn't until I learned to love myself that I met Mr. Right.

Tragically, though after being together for almost 3 ½ years, Brett was killed in an automobile accident. And the year after his death was the most challenging year of my life. I was devastated. It's really difficult to describe in words what I went through that year, and still give the experience justice. I felt like my world had stopped. You know, suddenly... all the things I bitched about before, like my job, like the traffic, like Brett not calling when he said he would...stupid stuff...it became so insignificant the day he died. Nothing mattered anymore My greatest fear had come to fruition. In my heart, there was nothing worse that could have happened, so I had nothing left to stress about...nothing left to be fearful of. I just felt...empty. I prayed for guidance, and I had to trust that God would take care of me, because I didn't know how to lead my life on my own anymore. It was all planned out before, and suddenly, in a moment it all changed. I was lost. So, I just surrendered my whole being into the hands of my Higher Power. I have often said that the year after Brett's death was the worst year of my life...and the best year of my life. I know, you're probably saying to yourself, "How could it have ever been the *best* year of your life?" Let me see if I can explain...

When I "Let go and Let God" that year, I had this clarity that I had never experienced before, and there was literally no more stress in my life. Yes, there was great sadness at that time...but no more worries. I believe that angels were surrounding me, guiding me, and helping me work through the grief. Because of this clarity, anything I wanted to know, the answers would come to me immediately. I was open to seeing whatever signs were given to me from the Heavens. For example, I asked God if Brett were still with me in spirit, only to wake the next morning "feeling" a squeezing in my hand as if he were holding it... Another example was the little wind chimes inside my apartment that would randomly chime every morning about the same time of day that he was killed; yet there were no windows open or air conditioner running...so virtually no wind to cause them to ring. There were a lot of strange, supernatural occurrences that I experienced that year... but there was one in particular that I'll never forget - I had a dream one night, about 2 months after Brett had passed away, that **I was** in a car accident. When I awoke from that dream, I recalled every detail of it, and still can to this very day:

My accident occurred on Route 27 in Maryland (in my dream)... I was in a head on collision, and immediately after the impact I was standing in a long, dark, narrow hallway. At the end of the hallway was a door, with a bright white light permeating the edges of the doorframe. I opened the door and walked into another hallway; this one was lit up very brightly. There were many doors in that corridor, but I decided to open the first one on the right hand side. I walked into a big room filled with music, laughter and lots of people, and over to the right of me was a table where Brett sat with two girls. He looked at me and said, "I've been waiting for you". He got up from the table, held my hand and walked me back out into the hallway, where we proceeded to go in through another doorway. The room we entered together was filled with guitars, hanging on the wall. He played several of them for me; each guitar had its own unique and beautiful sound. He told me that was his room, and that we each had our own special room. Next, he walked me down the hallway and opened up another door, where we entered "my room"! It was a lavish hotel suite with a cart with fancy food on it and in the bathroom was an oversized bathtub, filled with bubble bath. The dream ended with Brett and I making love.

Three days after having that dream, I was driving down *the real* Route 27 on a foggy morning –at the very spot where I had my "dream" accident – and a white horse came out of nowhere, walking down the road, towards my car. Because of the fog, I had been driving very cautiously that morning, and was able to slow down and come to a stop. The horse stopped too, facing me in front of my car. Then it turned away and ran down into the pasture, disappearing into the fog. Now remember, the horse was real. It wasn't a dream. But I saw the horse in

the same *exact* location that I had been in the "dream" accident. Okay…
so this story gets better. 3 days after seeing the horse, I was ***actually in***
a head on collision that was caused by a deer running out in the road.
And yes, you guessed it… it was in the same exact location on Route
27 where I had seen the horse only a few days prior, and the same exact
location where I had been in my "dream" accident. My car also caught
on fire and a looker-on called the fire department. But before the fire-
men got there, a bearded man came up to my car with a bucket of sand
and put the fire out, and then disappeared into the pasture, much like
the white horse did. I don't know exactly why this string of strange
events occurred. However, I don't believe that it was just coincidental.
Personally, I think it was a Divine wake-up call! My life changed that
year; it was the year that I deeply connected with my Higher Power,
and I learned that when you let go of the need to control and let go of
your fears, that everything in life becomes clearer. I felt like Brett had
been in my life for a reason, and after his death I made the decision
that since he could not physically be with me anymore, I would try to
adopt his beautiful and loving attitude as my own. I felt somehow that
doing so would keep his spirit alive. He was a positive influence in my
life and I wanted to carry on his spirit and be a positive influence in
others' lives. Now, more than ever I felt compelled to inspire people
and encourage them to be happy and live their dreams.

The year after his death was an interesting time. I let go of the
need to control everything. I did a lot of journal writing - I wrote
down thoughts, feelings, and questions. Eventually I wrote about
more than my feelings, and began writing about my desires. I wrote
in my journal that I wanted to meet somebody that I could love again
the way I had loved Brett. I was very specific on the details of this
person. It was important that he lived close to me and it wasn't a
long-distance relationship. I described him as a younger man with
blond hair and blue eyes. I wanted to meet somebody who was
adventurous, and who wanted to have children. I enjoyed having a

loving partner and I wrote in my journal that one day I wanted to be involved in a loving relationship again. About a year after Brett died, that man came into my life. His name is Todd and we've been married now for over 18 years.

After we married, Todd and I relocated to Florida and had a son. Shortly after the September 11th tragedy, when my son was a toddler and I was in my late 30's, I left the airline industry and started working in the Admissions Department of a private college. The school specialized in teaching students how to make films and other types of entertainment media. I wasn't exactly working on stage or television, but I guess you could say that my career was still related to the entertainment industry. My job as Admissions Representative was to recruit students into the school. The school provided an education to help people get into a career that many only dream about. When I first began my job, I thought it was so cool! Most of my day I listened to the needs of the students and identified if their goals matched up with the education that we provided, and if so, I would walk them through the enrollment process. I genuinely cared about these kids. Many of them had fears associated with going to college and with moving forward in pursuing their dream career. Some of those fears were based on financial and other obstacles that might make it harder to get into school. Some fears were based on moving away from home and getting out of their comfort zone. However, when it came down to it, one of the biggest fears my students faced was fear of failure at succeeding in *their* chosen field. That's irony! Here I was - a dropout from a performing arts school, and I had a career motivating students to pursue their dream of working in the entertainment and media field! I loved it. Dropping out of acting school was a choice I had made for myself, yet I still never doubted my ability to succeed at whatever I wanted in life.

Motivating those students was a perfect career fit for me. And probably the most fulfilling part of my job was seeing them graduate and become a success in their profession. But there were downsides to the work. For eight years I spent my life sitting at a desk for ten hours per day. I worked late into the night many times, and also on weekends. I hardly ever took a break. As the hours grew so did my butt. Life began to get out of my control, and I rarely saw my family because of the hours I put in. Both pressure and pounds piled on me. Now that I was in my early 40s, in a sedentary, stressful job, following the latest "diet of the week" just wouldn't take the weight off anymore. No matter what I did, I seemed to get fatter. The stress increased daily at work as well as at home. On top of the demands of the job, I still had a family and private life to manage, which meant attending my son's sporting events, spending time with my husband, grocery shopping, cleaning the house…you know, all that stuff that comes with being a wife and mother. I guess you *could* say that my life was good. Even though it was stressful, I had a good-paying job, a house, a healthy child, and a loving husband. I had a lot to be grateful for and I came to accept the way things were, including my weight. Then one day at work I started having chest pains and numbness in my arm. I had Todd drive me to the hospital and the doctor performed a heart-catheter procedure to see if there was any blockage. They kept me in the cardiac care unit for a week to run more tests. Fortunately, my heart was clear, although my cholesterol, triglycerides, and blood pressure were all very high. I was afraid, because I had heard that stress could kill people. Suddenly losing weight was no longer an issue of looking good, losing weight was going to be important for staying alive. Now you would think that would have been the catalyst that prompted my ultimate and permanent weight loss and the life changing program that this book is about. But it wasn't. It should have been, but it wasn't.

Two years later, I reached my highest weight ever, and had become even unhappier with the way things were going. Even though there were aspects of my job that I loved, it wasn't what I truly wanted to be doing for the rest of my life. Every day that I went to work I had to pump myself up in order to do my job well. I came to realize that I wanted more out of my life than what I was getting from my job: to have my own business, write a book, act in Community Theater, become a professional speaker, go out dancing, go camping, spend more time with my family. I wanted to be thin and feel freedom like I did when I was a child. I fantasized about being able to do a cartwheel again! I dreamed of being able to play with my son without getting worn out or being too tired. Instead of following any of my dreams, I was dedicating myself to my job, which ironically, was motivating others to follow their dreams. And that required working many hours of the week sitting in my chair, which resulted in me becoming obese. Because of my weight, I was totally disgusted with myself, and ashamed of my body. I didn't know who I was anymore. Depression engulfed me to the point that I didn't want to do anything outside of work and sleep. I didn't have the energy to regardless. Whenever there were work parties or functions, I never wanted to attend. I blamed my job for my appearance and my weight and for taking time away from my family. But it wasn't my job's fault. The fault was all mine. I had made everything and everyone else a priority over my own health. I hated the way I looked and I didn't want anybody to see me. I didn't want to dress up, and frankly I looked horrible in everything I put on. I didn't want to go to parties, or out to places with my husband, and the last thing I wanted to do was put on a bathing suit in front of anyone. (Let me tell you, Florida is not the place you want to live if you don't want to wear a bathing suit!) I was miserable. I started having a hard time remembering the things I was grateful for. It didn't help that I was in my early forties…I think I was having a mid-life crisis. My parents were aging and I was faced with the reality that I only have one life and it was getting shorter. Taking care of them really woke me up to my own mortality. Mom was in her eighties and was quite ill. She took a dozen different drugs just to feel halfway decent and to keep her body functioning. I loved my mom and hated seeing her this way, but the more I thought about it, if I kept going down this path of self-destruction, I would be in the same boat as her when I reached her age. That's if I made it that far! The way I was going I would be lucky to make it into my fifties. Then one day came when everything changed.

It was a typical hot, Florida weekend, and my husband and son wanted to go to the beach. I figured that there would be a million people at the beach and hoped I would just blend in with the crowd. Reluctantly I put on my bathing suit, packed us up, and we took off for the coast. Of course, as soon as we chose a spot on the beach, we ran into some old friends that we hadn't seen in ages. They ended up hanging around with us all day. That day was mortifying - I was at my heaviest weight ever, in a bathing suit, parading around in front of our old friends. If that wasn't bad enough, my husband took pictures that I looked at later that night. After seeing the pictures, I just went into my bedroom and cried. Here I was, successful in all other areas of my life - I had a job with a good income that allowed us to afford a few luxuries in life, a gorgeous husband who adored me, and an amazing son. So why was I fat? If I could be successful at everything else, then why wasn't I successful at weight loss? As I sobbed, I reached onto my bookshelf to find something to read to help ease my pain. I picked out a book called, Life's *Little Instruction Book*. I hadn't read it in many years. I opened the book and unintentionally turned directly to a page with a quote that said, "Judge your success by the degree that you're enjoying peace, health, and love". That was it. I guess I wasn't really that successful after all. It was then that I realized I was truly unhappy, no matter how great things appeared to be. Although I was grateful for what I had, my life was out of balance. And this reflected in the mirror, and in that photo from the day on the beach. It showed in my body, my face, and my eyes. I did a lot of soul searching that night and I remembered back to the time when

I was thin and healthy and felt sexy and desirable. Thinking back on it I was able to make a connection. I realized that the reason I had stayed thin for so many years in my twenties was not because I dieted and exercised, it was because I was truly happy and I loved myself. And more importantly, I believed that I was thin and was deserving of being thin. And the results of these feelings and thoughts about myself gave me the body and self-confidence I had dreamed of. Yet now, I was in a far different place emotionally. I knew that I needed to change my current, negative vicious circle into a positive one. If I wanted to bring back my inner Vixen, then I was going to have to start by changing the way I think.

I reluctantly returned to work after an eye-opening weekend. That afternoon I asked Allison to do a special project for me before she left for the evening. Being that she was a very loyal and dedicated assistant, I was a little surprised when she said that she couldn't help me out. She told me that she was scheduled to go to the gym for a class and she couldn't miss it. Immediately my interest piqued. *Maybe a gym membership is what I need,* I thought to myself. So I asked her where she worked out, which caused her to become very quiet and shy. She seemed almost embarrassed to tell me. After pressing her further, she reluctantly pulled up a website to show me her gym. I was shocked by what I saw! Allison was going to a pole-dance fitness class at a women's only, alternative fitness studio. How cool was that! After she left my office I shut the door so nobody could hear me, and I picked up the phone to make the call that literally changed my life. At my weight, I wasn't very comfortable with the idea of dancing on a pole in front of a bunch of other women, so I set up a private lesson for the following Saturday.

The girl on the phone was very helpful and sweet, but I thought I would die when she told me that the required workout attire would be short-shorts and high heels! Honestly, can you imagine a 210-pound woman in stilettos and short-shorts? However, I did as instructed and that private lesson turned out to be a pivotal moment in my life. To help set the mood for my lesson I brought in my Bon Jovi *Slippery When Wet* CD. It brought up great memories - the 80's were MY time! It was the decade when I was slim, single and sexy. In those days "hair metal" bands like Great White and Guns and Roses were at the top of the charts and when Tawney Kitaen was THE video vixen. So I thought it would help me loosen up if I had a few 80's tunes to rock out with! The lights dimmed down and the song went on, then I followed the instructor through the routine. After just a few minutes swinging around that pole and letting my hair down I had a sense of freedom that I hadn't felt in years. I looked in the mirror and didn't see the 210-pound girl that was in the beach photo earlier that week. I saw a beautiful, sensual woman that I hadn't seen in almost 15 years. It was an epiphany. The woman that I longed to be was staring at me right there in the mirror. She was my inner Vixen. And I did not want to let her go. After years of being last on my list of priorities, I made a decision to put myself first, and become the woman I desired to be. I quickly learned that the fat was only the symptom and the result of not loving and taking care of myself. Once I began unleashing my inner Vixen, the weight started coming off, and I set a plan in motion to fully become her. I started to dress like her, walk like her, talk like her, think like her and be the confident and sexy woman that I knew I was.

I am no longer an Admissions Representative, now I am the co-owner of a women's fitness studio in Orlando, Florida, and a motivational speaker who travels the country inspiring women to be empowered and change their lives. My life has turned around completely, and with the *Vixen Unleashed* program I am going to show you how to do the same! If you are tired of settling for last place on your to-do list, join me for the ride of your life on Interstate Vixen12, where we will discover how to get your life, your body and your sexy back once and for all!

Chapter 2

Rules of the Road

Afew months before Brett died he ordered a set of motivational cassette tapes from a TV infomercial. After he passed away I packed a lot of his personal items in a box, including the unopened cassettes and buried them in my closet. It wasn't until I started my career as an Admissions Representative that I dug them out and listened to them. I found that the messages on the tapes were nearly identical to the messages that I was giving my students! The program was simple - If you think it, you can achieve it. Act as if you have it now, and take actions that move you towards that vision. Believe in yourself and believe in your dreams, and you will succeed.

By listening to those tapes, I discovered that there is actually a systematic method to achieving your goals; I was fascinated by what I was hearing! Throughout my career as an Admissions Representative, I went on to read and listen to tons of books and CDs related to motivation, and the subconscious mind, to enable me to better serve my students. I learned from motivational speakers like Tony Robbins and Dr. Wayne Dyer. Their programs became my "mentors", and their strategies for success became my "bible". It became an obsession to learn as much as I could about how the mind worked. It was amazing to learn how, by tapping into our subconscious, we can dissolve negative core beliefs about ourselves and exchange them for positive ones. Through changing our early negative conditioning, we can literally design our destiny in life. I used these principals in my former career as an Admissions Representative. My students connected with me and I made a difference in their outlook on life! I realized I had a gift for motivating people to have self-belief, and achieve their dreams and goals. When my career path and my life took a new direction, I used the same principals for success along with my knowledge of health and fitness, to design *Vixen Unleashed*, which is the program you are about to experience.

SLIGHT CHANGE IN COURSE

Starting any new program can be intimidating. *"I have to eat right, exercise, change the way I think and do it all right now? Maybe next year! "* But a successful program does not have to include torture or grand sweeping changes. One of the secrets I have learned through my years of studying the techniques of truly successful people - those who have achieved great wealth, prestige, personal satisfaction, and flourishing relationships – is the discipline of making small changes that compound into great gains. Analyzing the lives and habits of these individuals shows the things they have in common: they use their time mindfully, they set attainable daily; weekly and monthly goals; they chart a path and stick to it. They recognize that investing a little bit each day, will not only lead to the ROI (return on investment) that you desire, but it will keep you from getting overwhelmed and quitting.

This is not a new theory! Think about those old adages: The journey of 1000 miles begins with a single step. Or this one: How do you eat an elephant? Answer: one bite at a time! This program is about making small, smart choices, repeatedly over time to change habits, and to progress you toward your goal. If you practice good habits consistently day in and day out, you will achieve the vision you have for yourself, and surpass others who did not have the insight to chart a course and follow it to its completion.

And where is our course taking us? From your Comfort Zone to Freedom, where you will be the woman you always dreamed to become! You have to take the risk, and leave your comfort zone if you want to make this change. Once you put your sports car on the road, the only reason to look in your rear-view mirror is to see the dust you've left behind. This is a one-way trip and there is no going back!

The program that follows is one that I tested and perfected on myself and on others who have had great success at losing the weight, changing their thinking and embracing the sensual, beautiful women they authentically are. I am so pleased and excited to share with you how I made this transformation, and to be your guide on this incredible journey. You will see why the *Vixen Unleashed* program is so different than others, because it addresses your whole woman – body, mind and spirit!

This 12-week journey is designed in a particular sequence to maximize your potential. You are not going to be changing who you are; you're simply going to become a better version of you! You will be learning about your inner and outer self, following a solid eating plan, and easing into an exercise program that will eventually become as much as a part of your daily routine as taking a shower. You will learn to undo years of negative programming, while laughing and having fun in the process!

Each week will teach you a new concept, and will end at a Mile Marker where you'll be given a set of action steps to complete before going on to the next week. Throughout this journey you will be learning new skills, and tossing out the baggage of negative thoughts, behavior and excess weight. I suggest that you read ahead through the entire book first. Then, I urge you to go back and re-read each week in the program, follow the instructions in your action steps at each Mile Marker, and incorporate these changes, *one week at a time*. That way, you can integrate these new thoughts and behaviors incrementally, and the new thinking patterns and life-style changes can take root in you. As we continue down Interstate Vixen12, you will see how the assignments build off one another, to create long lasting change. I encourage you to purchase a small journal that you can put into your purse, diaper bag or briefcase. Use it to track your weight, diet, exercise, thoughts and feelings. Keeping a record of those times when you may struggle will allow you to spot patterns in feelings or situations that cause you to turn to food. Also, reading over your goals you've listed for yourself will reinforce your vision. Tracking is a proven method that forces you to be conscious of your decisions and choices. Do not neglect to track, it is a small but extremely important habit. And just like any good road trip, *Vixen Unleashed* will also be more fun when you do it with a friend. So before you begin, I encourage you to invite a friend to share the adventure with you.

I am so happy to be able to take you on this journey. If you remember, my desire to be on stage or in the soaps factored highly into my childhood dreams. I may have never made it as a soap star, but where the Universe has guided me is even better. I have been able to take my passion for the stage and marry it with my gift for speaking and motivating others. I have always been a dreamer, and now I am blessed to teach you to be one as well – to dream big, set a course, and reach your goal! Every woman has a beautiful soul that is her true inner "sexy". But sometimes that soul gets a little lost in this world. If you have the willingness to do the work and the desire to change your life and make a better version of YOU, then hop into your convertible - it's time to leave the Comfort Zone. We're going on a road trip that will lead you to good health, more energy, and a body that is reflective of your true inner Vixen!

Chapter 3

Your Fuel Gauge

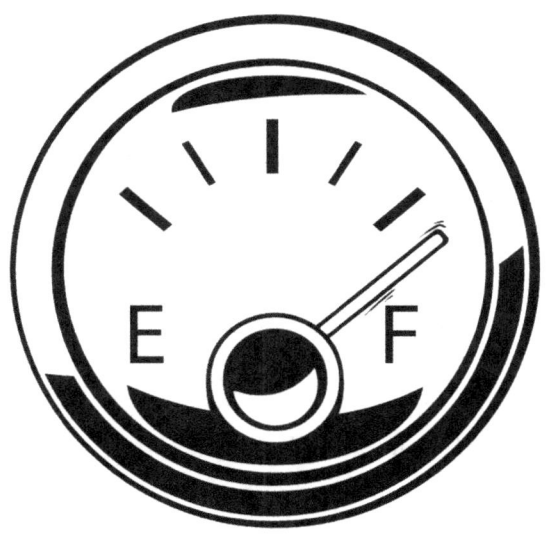

Before taking off on a road trip, it's always good to take your car into a trusted mechanic to ensure everything is in proper working order. I used to have a 1991 Jaguar XJS (with a V12 engine, of course!) and I generally took it to a Jaguar specialist, but once I took it to a general mechanic for an issue I was experiencing with the car. To make a long story short, they were unfamiliar with this unique machine and couldn't seem to diagnose the problem, much less fix it. I learned then, the importance of always going to a specialist who fully understood how to work on my specific automobile. The same principle applies to your body. When it comes to your health, its important to go to a medical provider who looks at the whole picture and not just the symptoms. A functional medicine practitioner does just that – they work together with you to figure out, and get rid of the cause, rather than just mask the symptoms. Going to a functional medicine practitioner is like taking your car to an auto specialist who knows your particular vehicle, and understands its idiosyncrasies. You may have never heard of functional medicine before, or you may not know what it has to do with losing weight. If so, allow me to help. The Institute for Functional Medicine defines functional medicine like this:

"Functional medicine addresses the underlying causes of disease, using a systems-oriented approach and engaging both patient and practitioner in a therapeutic partnership. It is an evolution in the practice of medicine that better addresses the healthcare needs of the 21st century. By shifting the traditional disease-centered focus of medical practice to a more patient-centered approach, functional medicine addresses the whole person, not just an isolated set of symptoms. Functional medicine practitioners spend time with their patients, listening to their histories and looking at the interactions among genetic, environmental, and lifestyle factors that can influence long-term health and complex, chronic disease. In this way, functional medicine supports the unique expression of health and vitality for each individual."

This is important when talking about weight loss because you are an individual with individual body issues and an individual body type. So when looking for a good medical provider, you want someone who knows how to test your hormones, your adrenal glands, your thyroid, your genetics, your cardiac status, your gastro-intestinal health and can recognize patterns of behavior that might lead to self-sabotage along the way. You want a specialist. I specialize in blending the elements of fitness, nutrition and introspection to help women create healthier bodies and lead dynamic and passionate lives; I'm also a food psychology coach. For your road trip on Interstate Vixen 12, I have teamed up with several other specialists in their fields in order to bring you the very best program, possible. Your nutrition specialist for the *High Octane Diet* will be Dr. Keesha Ewers. Dr. Keesha is an Advanced Registered Nurse Practitioner who has decades of experience in functional medicine and in getting to the root of imbalance, illness, and weight issues. You can read more about her at www.vixenunleashed.com .

When preparing for your road trip, you will need to know how to fuel and care for your car for optimum performance. Just like every car is not the same, no two humans are exactly alike. This is why there isn't really a "one-size fits all" diet. With all the diets available to us, how do you decide what is right for you? When your car breaks down and you take it to a mechanic, they have to run diagnostic tests to see what the problem is before they try to fix it. The same applies to people. A good functional medicine specialist will run the appropriate diagnostic tests to see what's happening with your body. Based on the results of these tests, the specialist would then outline a very specific course for you to follow. Here are some of the most helpful tests that he or she would use to help determine your diet plan:

- Hormone testing
- Checking for Insulin Resistance
- Thyroid function
- Allergy testing
- ApoE genetic testing
- Inflammation
- Energy transport
- Heavy metal testing
- Detoxification pathways
- Digestion

I want to stress that you DO NOT have to have all of these tests run, in order to start your weight loss program. Here is why - In the *Vixen Unleashed* program you will begin by giving up sugar, foods with gluten, and most processed foods. These are commonly the foods that women reach for when reacting to stress and negative emotions. And unfortunately, they are also the ones that typically do the most harm to your body and are the most physically addictive. Gluten, a popular weight-loss buzzword these days, is a protein that's found primarily in wheat and wheat flour. However it's also found in oats and barley and many other processed foods. It has been linked to everything from chronic sinusitis to depression to gastrointestinal disorders and more. By eliminating gluten and sugar from your diet, which are some of the biggest culprits in the obesity epidemic, and then reintroducing them later, you are essentially doing *your own self-testing*, at a very basic level, to determine your dietary needs. Once you get these common toxins out of your body, when you reintroduce them, you should know almost immediately how well YOUR body tolerates them and whether you can enjoy them in small amounts, on occasion, or not at all. Throughout this program, we will also be working on changing your impulses to eat processed carbohydrates as a reaction to stressful situations. We will be diving deep into the psyche to turn around long-standing behaviors and conditioning to help you change your thoughts, change your choices, and ultimately change your habits, so that by the time you've reached your health goals, you're less likely to gain the weight back. You're also going to be learning how to listen to your body and understand what it needs to thrive. By the time you are done with the 12 weeks, you will be very much in tune with your own body and will have a pretty good idea of what works for you, and what doesn't.

However, for a more accurate reading of what you should be eating to maintain optimal health, it's not a bad idea to get the testing done with a functional medicine practitioner before beginning your diet program. Keep in mind that the money you spend on those tests upfront can quite possibly mean less money spent in the future on doctors' visits, prescriptions, and hospital bills. If you are interested in having these tests run, and you don't have access to a practitioner of functional medicine in your area, Dr. Keesha can help. Her contact information can be found at www.vixenunleashed.com .

When developing the *High Octane Diet* for the *Vixen Unleashed* program, I called my friend, Dr. Keesha to get some advice. With her expertise in nutrition and functional medicine, and mine as a food psychology coach, together we came up with the perfect formula! This diet is healthy and balanced, and is based on what has worked for my body, current scientific evidence, Dr. Keesha's advice, and the advice of my doctor almost thirty years ago…

When I was around 20 years old, I decided to become a vegetarian. I lived in Asheville, NC and there seemed to be a lot of vegetarians who lived there. It was kind of the "in" thing to do at the time… And, I needed to lose a few pounds, so I thought I'd give it a shot. After all - all the vegetarians I knew were skinny! Veganism and vegetarianism can definitely be a healthy way to eat, as long as you're doing it correctly (and for the right body-type). What I didn't realize is that vegetarians have to be diligent about eating properly to make sure they are getting adequate calories, protein and vitamins. You can't just binge on bread and expect that your body will be healthy!

So, one evening, about three weeks after starting my new vegetarian diet, I was out to dinner at a Japanese hibachi-style restaurant with a group of my friends. Soon after we ordered dinner, I left to go to the ladies room. On the return trip to my table, the lights started closing in on me and I began experiencing tunnel vision. Before I knew it, I fainted! It was the only time in my life that had ever happened to me. After seeing the doctor and having blood work done, I discovered that I was hypoglycemic. The way I had been eating had caused my blood sugar to be unstable, which inevitably caused the fainting episode. He gave me this advice: eat 5-6 small meals each day and include a little bit of protein in each meal. Simple. And kind of revolutionary if you remember that it was almost 30 years ago. He told me that if I kept a constant stream of balanced calories coming into my body throughout the day I'd neither experience the spikes in insulin (leading to the inevitable crash and burn… or, in my case, passing out!) nor get famished and then make terrible choices based on extreme hunger. So when I came to that pivotal moment in my life where I was ready to make real changes in my health, I decided to implement that same simple eating strategy that my doctor had prescribed to me so many years before.

The foundational principals of the nutrition portion of this program are based off of my own personal experience with weight loss; eating 5-6 times per day, enjoying a colorful variety of fruits and vegetables, and incorporating a little protein and healthy fat into each small meal. Simple. Protein is a denser source of calories that slows digestion. It will keep you fuller longer and has a zero effect on our insulin levels. Colorful fruits and vegetables contain all of the micronutrients you need to stay healthy, fight off infection, and live to be a little old lady. Healthy fats such as those found in nuts, seeds, and mono-unsaturated oils, keep you satisfied, your joints lubricated, your skin glowing, and your brain functioning properly. Our bodies need fat to not only to survive, but also to thrive. These three elements together are a powerful combination. When in doubt, eat lean protein, a plentitude of colorful fruits and vegetables, and healthy fats.

SUGAR IN YOUR TANK

The American Nutrition Association reported on a talk given by three well-respected doctors back in 1996.[1] The doctors questioned why the rates of obesity have climbed, while the rates of dietary fat consumption have fallen dramatically. They hypothesized that carbohydrates were to blame, explaining that blood glucose is increased by carbohydrates and stimulates insulin production, which then stores the glucose (sugar) as fat. All carbohydrates produce an insulin response, some more than others – the more refined (think white flours, pastas, white rice, potatoes, sugars) the larger the insulin dose your pancreas has to release to get the blood sugar volume under control. If you chronically overeat highly refined carbohydrates, your body can become resistant to the insulin. This is called insulin resistance [2], and soon your body will produce more and more insulin to deal with the influx of carbohydrates. The more insulin you produce, the more sugar is stored as fat instead of being used for energy. And the best way to thwart it is to remove high glycemic index carbs from your diet, which are the ones that will tend to spike your insulin. Carbohydrates that have a low glycemic index are those that do not spike your insulin as dramatically. These include brown rice, whole grains (like barley, quinoa, oats), whole-wheat pastas and breads, beans, etc. Low GI carbs are the only way to go. A useful Glycemic Index chart can be found at: www. glycemicedge.com.

As you're following this program, you might be pleasantly surprised to know that the reason you've had such difficulty losing

---

1   Sears, Gerdes, Juetersonke *NOHA NEWS*, Summer 1997

2   Anne W Thorburn (1989). "Fructose-induced in vivo insulin resistance and elevated plasma triglyceride levels in rats". *American Journal of Clinical Nutrition*.

weight in the past has NOTHING to do with your lack of willpower. The problem is not that women lack willpower, or lack the desire to lose weight. The problem is that they have sugar rampaging through their bodies, acting like an addictive drug. And no matter what kind of "willpower" a woman may have, until they get this addictive "drug" out of their system, they simply CANNOT fight it! You see, it's not that you can't stop eating it simply because it tastes so good. Sugar also affects our brain chemistry. In 2002, research at Princeton University showed that sweets activated the brains beta-endorphin receptor cites, the same cites that are excited by an intake of heroin or morphine [3] Then later, in 2008 a panel studied the effects of sugar and found it caused the release of dopamine in the brain, and determined sugars to have addictive potential, with symptoms of craving, withdrawal, and binging — similar to the process that occurs in drug addiction. [4]

So, because of its addictive nature, without first removing excess sugar from your diet, you can see why it's impossible to create the lifelong changes you desire. It's not that you don't have willpower. It's that you have SUGAR coursing through your veins! In the *Vixen Unleashed* program, we initially remove added sugar, gluten and processed foods to stop the physical addiction, and give you the time (10 weeks) you need to address and work through the deeper, psychological desire to medicate your feelings with those same foods. Once you have learned the skills to effectively manage your choices, then we reintroduce gluten back into your body. After being without it for 10 weeks, it won't take long for you to recognize whether or not your body is gluten sensitive. And eventually, you can decide for yourself if you want to reintroduce processed sugar or other "junk-food". For

---

3   Avena, Bocarsly, Rada, Kim and Hoebel, unpublished, http://www.ncbi. nlm.nih.gov/pubmed/12055324

4   Princeton.edu top stories — Dec. 10 2008 - http://www.princeton.edu/ main/news/archive/S22/88/56G31/index.xml?section=topstories

now, you'll be getting your "sweet" fix via natural sources. Foods such as fruits and dairy have natural sugars in them, which you'll be consuming in the *High Octane Diet*. We limit those foods, however to help you stay at a lower amount of daily sugar intake throughout your program, and help reduce those cravings for the more addictive stuff. I recommend that you try to eat the fruits and dairy that have lower sugar content more often, and ones with higher sugar content less frequently. I've notated which ones are lower in sugar content in your *High Octane Diet* food list.

Once you've learned how to overcome impulses to eat as a reaction to stress, and you have reached your goals, I firmly believe that you can enjoy anything in moderation, or on special occasion, unless you discover that you have a severe sensitivity of some sort. Although, it is highly likely that by the time we re-introduce these foods back into your diet, you won't want them simply because you'll know how good it feels to live without them! Within just a few short weeks, your desire to eat cookies and ice cream will practically vanish. And once you get these possible toxins out of your body, I promise that it will be much easier to say "no". And, if you really want to shoot for optimal health, and not just weight loss… you may end up opting to never eat sugar or wheat again. That will be *your* choice, but you don't have to make that decision right now. For the first 10 weeks, you will be consuming foods in a more natural state.

For now, you will still be eating carbohydrates from sources like legumes, nuts, colorful non-starchy vegetables, some starchy veggies and some grains, and minimal amounts of dairy, but it is likely you'll be eating far less than what you are used to. Initially, for a few days you may have headaches and other side effects from removing this stuff from your diet. If you begin to experience anything like this, I recommend adding an extra piece of fruit each day during the first week (if needed) to help decrease those side effects. When those sugar cravings sneak up, I'd rather you grab an apple with sugar-free natural peanut butter on it, than see you devour a candy bar. Then, by week two, make sure that you're eating no more than the recommended amounts of fruit servings per day, according to your chart. I also do not recommend chemical sweeteners such as aspartame or Splenda. Instead, try a plant derivative like stevia or a small amount of agave nectar in your coffee, which has a lower impact on your insulin. In addition, throughout the program you'll also be striving for 8-10 glasses of water per day, being sure to stay well hydrated.

When you are ready to begin your program, the next chapter will walk you through the *High Octane Diet*, which offers a great food list for you to work from. Instead of thinking about what things you can't eat, try focusing on what you can eat and enjoy! Grocery shopping will be streamlined since you will be shopping almost exclusively on the perimeter of the store, where all of the fresh foods are kept. The only real reason to venture to the center aisle is for your nuts, oils and vinegars, nut butters, condiments and spices and perhaps occasionally for a few of the allowed whole-grains. Use this list to create meal ideas for yourself by combining items that suit your personal tastes. I recommend planning and writing out your meals/snacks for a week, and post this daily meal list where you can easily see it, like on your refrigerator. It will help make grocery shopping easier, and help you stick to your eating plan.

Now that you know the basic foods you'll be eliminating in the *Vixen Unleashed* program, and why you're eliminating them, it's time to get on to the good stuff! In the next chapter you'll be learning about all of the amazing foods that you *can* eat, how much you should eat for your body and your goals, and a simpler way for you to make those healthier choices, rather than counting calories, carbs or fat grams. Initially, it will take some weighing, measuring, tracking, practice and patience. But before long it will become second nature and you will start seeing the pounds melt away!

Chapter 4

The High Octane Diet

(This diet can be modified to fit various dietary needs and caloric intake requirements)

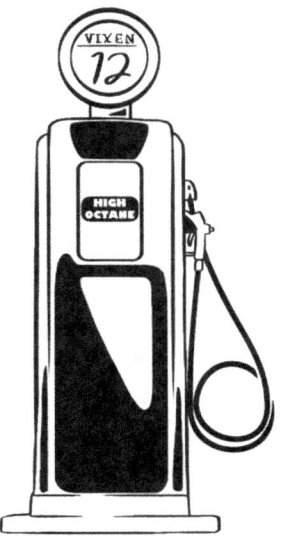

If you've ever gone to a gas station and filled your tank, you've probably noticed that there are several different grades of fuel to choose from. Premium grades of fuel are ones that are higher in octane. When using premium fuel, you'll get better performance out of your car. And so it is with the fuel we put into our bodies... The more superior quality of food we eat, the better performance we get out of our bodies.

The High Octane Diet will give your body the quality fuel it needs, in just the right amounts for you to thrive; giving you increased energy level, mental clarity, and better overall health. You'll notice in this food list, that there is a specific "grade" noted for each food source. The "grade" system is simply a way to put a value on the (amount of) food you eat. For example, 1 oz of chicken has a value of 1 grade of lean, quality protein. Therefore, 3 oz of chicken = 3 grades of protein. And ½ cup of cottage cheese has a value of 1 grade of protein. So, 1 cup of cottage cheese = 2 grades of protein. Make sense?

Ideally, whenever possible, I recommend that you choose foods that are organic and non-GMO, and animal proteins which are grass fed (beef), free-range (poultry), and antibiotic and hormone free. When buying premium foods, just like the fuel you put into your car, the better quality of fuel, often times means higher prices. And in some areas of the world, it is more difficult to find these higher qualities of foods. So this may not always be an option for everyone. This is not a requirement for your diet... but it is definitely _ideal,_ especially if you aim to gain optimal health, in addition to losing weight. So, any time that you can, I do recommend trying to opt for more natural and organic selections, free of pesticides and other chemicals. In the long run you're your body will thank you. Check at a local farmer's market, where many times you'll find those healthier choices at more reasonable prices... and of course, watch for sales in your local grocery store. Keep in mind that you won't be eating as much food, nor will you be eating the junk food that you have been up until now. Where you'll be spending a little more money on organic vegetables and free-range chicken, you'll be saving it by not buying ice cream, cookies, and those larger quantities of meats and other foods. In reality, when I started eating healthier to lose weight, I ended up saving about $20 per week, due to lowering the quantity of food I was eating, and getting rid of the costly junk food.

Next is a list of foods that you will be eating in the *High Octane Diet*. You'll notice that beside some of these foods, there is an (HF) notated. Also, certain fruits and dairy products have an asterisk (*) in front of them. The *asterisk indicates fruits and dairy products that are lower in sugar. The "HF" indicates which foods are higher in fiber. Fiber plays an important role in a healthy digestive system and helps lower your risk of colon cancer and heart disease. Fiber also helps reduce risks of obesity and obesity related diseases. You will want to make sure that you include several of the higher fiber foods into your daily meals and snacks.

Vegetables -1 Grade = ½ cup cooked or 1 cup raw

Artichoke hearts (HF)	Collard Greens (HF)	Okra
Asparagus	Chard/Swiss Chard	Onions
Bamboo shoots	(HF)	Peppers
Bean sprouts	Cucumbers	Radishes
Bell peppers	Eggplant	Shallots
Broccoli (HF)	Green beans (HF)	Spinach
Brussels sprouts (HF)	Kale (HF)	Summer squash
Cabbage (HF)	Leeks	Tomato
Cauliflower (HF)	Lettuce	Turnip Greens
Celery	Mushrooms	Turnips (HF)

Starches - 1 Grade =

1 c	Acorn squash (HF)	½ c	Buckwheat/Kasha (HF)
1/3 c	Amaranth	1 c	Winter Squash (HF)
1 c	Beets	½ c	Carrots
1/3 c	Brown Rice	½ c	Corn
1/3 c	Wild Rice	½	Corn on the cob

½ c Millet

1/3 c Quinoa (HF)

½ c Parsnip

2 Rice cakes – from brown rice

½ c Peas (green/English)

½ c Plantain

3-4 Rice crackers – from brown rice

½ c Potato (HF)

½ c Pumpkin

1/3 c Rice noodles – from brown rice

3 c Popcorn

1 c Snow peas

1/3 c Rice pasta – from brown rice

1 c Sweet potato

Fruits (no sugar added) 1 Grade =

1sm *Apple (HF)	1 *Kiwi (HF)	2 sm *Plums
4 Apricots-fresh	½ sm Mango	1 sm Pomegranate
½ *Banana med (HF)	1 c *Melon	3 Prunes med.
¾ c*Blackberries (HF)	1 sm Nectarine	2 T Raisins
¾ c *Blueberries (HF)	1 sm Orange	1 c *Raspberries (HF)
3 Dates or figs (HF)	1 c Papaya	1 ¼ c*Strawberries (HF)
½ c *Grapefruit (HF)	1 sm *Peach	2 Tangerines
15 Grapes	1 sm Pear (HF)	2 T Dried fruit
	¾ c *Pineapple	

Fats -1 Grade =

Limit fats that are underlined to no more than 1 or 2 grades per day

16	Pistachios	4	Pecan halves
10	Peanuts	4	Walnut halves
6	Almonds	2	Brazil nuts
6	Cashews	3 T	Coconut (unsweetened) (HF)
6	Mixed nuts		
5	Hazelnuts	2 T	Flax seed (ground) (HF)

2 T Chia seeds (ground) (HF)

2 T   Avocado (HF)

2 T   Half and Half

1 T   Pine nuts

1 T   Pumpkin seeds

1 T   Sesame seeds

1 T   Parmesan cheese

1 T   Sunflower seed kernels

1 T   Salad dressing w/quality oils

½ T   Nut butters

1 t   Butter

1 t   Mayonnaise

1 oz   85% Cocoa Chocolate

1 t   Oils: Almond, Canola (non-GMO), Coconut (virgin), Grape seed oil, Flax Seed Oil (cold pressed), Olive oil, Safflower & Sunflower

PROTEIN (choose leaner cuts) - 1 Grade =

1 oz – Chicken (skinless)

1 oz - Turkey (skinless)

1 oz - Beef

1 oz - Buffalo

1 oz - Lamb

1 oz – Wild Game

1 oz – Pork

1 oz - Tuna Fish

1 oz – Salmon

1 oz – Tilapia or White Fish

1 oz - Grouper

1 oz - Shell Fish

1 oz - Low Fat or Part Skim Mozzarella Cheese

1 oz – Low Fat Cheese

1 oz – Feta Cheese

1 oz – Veggie Burger

1 oz – Soy Burger

½ oz – Beef Jerky (very little to no sugar added)

1 – Whole Egg

2 – Egg Whites

2 – Sardines

1 c - Chili made with meat/beans

½ c – Tofu

½ c - Tempeh

½ c Black-Eyed Peas

½ c Pinto Beans

½ c Black Beans

½ c Kidney Beans

½ c   Edamame, steamed or boiled

½ c Lentils

1/3 c - Hummus

¼ cup - Natto

¼ cup – Cottage Cheese

¼ cup – Ricotta Cheese

½ scoop – Protein Powder

Dairy – 1 Grade =

8 oz   *Buttermilk, Nonfat or 1%

8 oz   *Cow's Milk – Nonfat,

Skim or 1%

8 oz   Plain Yogurt, Nonfat or 1%

8 oz *Unsweetened Chocolate or

Plain Almond Milk

4 oz   *Plain Greek Yogurt, Nonfat

or 1%

Each dairy grade counts as both a dairy and a protein grade (except for almond milk)

Number of Grades per Day per Calorie Level

Calorie Level	1200	1300	1400	1500	1600	1800	2000	2500
Lean Protein	11	11	12	13	14	15	17	22
Fats	5	6	6	8	8	9	10	11
Vegetables	4+	4+	4+	4+	4+	4+	5+	5+
Fruit	1	1	1	1	1	1	1	2
Starches	1	1	1	1	2	2	2	2
Dairy / Alt.	1	2	2	2	2	3	3	3

In the next chapter, you'll be learning how to determine your optimal fuel tank level (how many calories your body needs to lose weight). Once you've done this, then come back and refer to the *High Octane Diet* "grades" chart above to determine exactly how many "grades" you will need from each food-source category, based on your daily caloric goal. You can also find a grades chart at <u>www.vixenunleashed.com</u> .

Food grades are not all equal when it comes to calories. For example, 1 grade of lean beef will be slightly higher in calories than 1 grade of chicken breast. However, I do NOT want you counting calories in this program. I simply want you to determine your daily caloric goal (in the next chapter), and then just focus on sticking with your specified amount of grades within your calorie column. I want to help you reduce the stress in your life, so that your body will assimilate and digest food better, and you will drop the weight more easily. So, I don't want you worried about counting every little calorie, or stressed about eating 1258 calories one day when you're goal is 1200. This is NOT the point. Your body will adjust. Where you might overdo it one day because you ate a steak, another day you'll be eating fish and your number will probably go lower than your optimal caloric daily goal. Or there might be a day that you exercise more than usual and burn more calories, and another day that you do very little. Remember… it's about BALANCE. Trusting your instinct (feminine) will be just as important as calculating and following a rigid chart (masculine).

Here is an example to help you better understand how to count your food grades, especially when one food source is tracked in two separate category counts:

3 oz of chicken, ½ cup Greek yogurt, 6 pecans, and ½ cup of peaches are tracked as —

4 grades of protein - (3 oz of chicken plus ½ cup Greek yogurt - the yogurt counts as both a protein and a dairy)

1 grade of fruit - (1/2 cup peaches)

Special Considerations

- Include protein and fat in every meal and snack.
- Nuts and nut butters are high in protein, and although they should **not** be counted as a protein grade, it would not be necessary to include a protein grade with a snack that included nuts or nut butters, unless you just wanted to. (For example – an apple with sugar free peanut butter would be a balanced snack, even without added protein)
- Food allergies – If you have a known food allergy, do NOT eat those foods!
- For vegetarians, make sure to choose proteins that are plant based.
- Try to include at least one type of legume as 1 of your daily protein grades.
- Try to include nuts or nut-oils for at least 3 or 4 of your daily fat grades.
- Dairy is high in protein. So, be sure to include your dairy grade in both your total protein count **and** your total dairy count each day.
- The more (non-starch) vegetables you eat, the easier the weight will come off. They add fiber and micronutrients that are necessary to good health.
- Do **not** eat fruit by itself. Always choose a protein or higher protein fat, like nuts or nut butters to eat with it.

1 grade of fat - (the pecans)

1 grade of dairy - (½ cup of plain Greek yogurt)

For an easy way to help you track your progress, go to: <u>www. vixenunleashed.com</u>

Once you reach Week 11 of the program, we will reintroduce wheat and other foods with gluten. If you already know that you are wheat or gluten sensitive, or you've done the laboratory work and your individual body type determines that you should limit these foods, then remember, it's not mandatory to reintroduce them in Week 11. It's simply an option. On the same token, if you've had lab work done and it has shown that your body type tolerates and/or does well with wheat, you can include whole grain wheat and gluten products in your diet now, as long as you track them as a starch.

STAYING ON THE TRACK

I always recommend, for at least the first month that you are very careful to measure everything you eat. It might be a pain to begin with… but this is how you really get to know true portion sizes. It's SO easy to get off track when you are just assuming that you're eating the correct portion sizes. You can go on for weeks eating healthy foods and find yourself not losing weight, from something as simple as you not estimating your portions correctly. However, as you track your grades by weighing and measuring your food, you will begin to see what a serving size of protein, vegetables, or dairy looks like, and soon you can use other "handy" ways to measure your food, too. For example:

3-4 oz of meat (which would be 3-4 grades of protein) will be the size of the palm of your hand; 1 grade of cooked vegetables is the size of your fist, and 1 grade of salad or raw veggies is the size of "two fists"; 1 grade of fruit is the size of a tennis ball; 1 grade of cheese is about the size of your thumb; 1 grade of nut butter or olive oil is about the size of a ping-pong ball; 1 grade of nuts is about 6 nuts, so a handful of nuts will equate to 4 grades of fat.

In time you will be able to eat out at restaurants or as a guest in someone's home and estimate the proper portions for yourself based on these visual cues. But I urge you to measure and weigh, to really get an understanding of a true portion size at least for the first month. The other piece of advice I will give you to help you get your portions under control from the very beginning, is to pack your lunch and 2 snacks at the beginning of each day, whether you are going out for the day or staying home.

Eating small meals throughout the day, about every three hours, requires advanced planning. Having foods at the ready to grab and go, or take to work, will prevent you from skipping a meal and growing famished or grabbing a frozen yogurt at the mall instead. Precooking a large batch of chicken breasts, having nuts or berries packaged into individual serving sizes, fresh vegetables washed and cut for munching – will allow you to grab something healthy on the go to take with you. There are containers that are just perfect for the sizes you need. You'll find containers that are perfectly ¼ cup, ½ cup and 1 cup... as well as some that break it down even further. Fit and Fresh (http://fit-fresh.com/) containers are some of my favorites because they actually have markings on them, like a built in measuring cup. They also have some pretty sassy lunch bags! There are all kinds of cool travel food storage containers these days, with built in freezer pouches, which makes it easy to just throw them into your purse on your way out the door. I can't stress this enough – PLAN AHEAD, so you don't make a poor choice.

I want you to dedicate the first month of this program to packing daily, as many meals as you can in pre-portioned containers, making sure that you weigh your grades of protein before packing them. As you lay out your daily meals I want to make sure that you start your day off right by eating shortly after you get up in the morning. It will kick-start your metabolism and keep you from getting hungry and cranky later. You should also structure your exercise sessions in such a way that you take one of those meals within a half an hour after you are done.

Tracking your food is also a big key to this program. It will be important to track *how much* you eat, by tallying up your grades in each food category. However, it's equally important to write down *what* you eat in your journal. It will help you to pinpoint times of mindless or emotional eating, it will keep you honest about what exactly you are putting in your mouth, and make you think twice before consuming something that wasn't on your eating plan for that day – causing you to ask yourself, "do I really want to write this down?" I always liked to take it a step further and plan my daily meals on paper, writing down what I would eat for my 5 meals in one column, and in an adjacent column writing down what I actually ate to see where, how or why I might have deviated from my plan. Track carefully, daily and religiously and you will begin to see patterns in your eating behavior, which will help you in the internal motivation work we'll be doing in future chapters.

Sensual Eating

Recently I joined a group of girlfriends in Sedona Arizona for a retreat. We hadn't seen each other in a while. After hiking to one of the vortexes to experience some spiritual rejuvenation, we decided to grab a bite to eat. We found this quaint little restaurant that was situated right beside of a stream, where the gorgeous red rock mountains were jutting up behind it. After hiking all morning in the Arizona heat, we were all hot and sweaty and excited to find comfort in the air-conditioned café. Our server sat us at a table near a window so we could see the beautiful scenery while we had lunch. I ordered a cold iced-tea and a large colorful salad with grilled salmon on top of it. As I sat there and ate the salad and drank my tea, I felt like I was on another planet! The experience was so amazing!! I found myself just relaxing and feeling the cool air, enjoying the conversation between good friends, and eating my food as if I had never had tasted food before! I savored each and every bite, and imagined the veggies and healthy fat in the salmon nourishing my body. And as I felt each sip of iced-tea go down my throat, I closed my eyes and visualized it hydrating my entire body. I laugh about the experience now, because I just know I must have looked like I was having a "food" orgasm! What must these girls have thought? I was simply experiencing sensual eating! As you are going through the *Vixen Unleashed* program, try to make a conscious effort to eat more *sensually*. Take a moment of silence, and take a few deep breaths before each meal to relax your body and mind, and be grateful for the food you will be eating. Then slow down, and savor each moment and each bite of food, and enjoy your surroundings!

In a nutshell:

What:

- Choose a variety of colorful vegetables and fruits – think of eating a daily rainbow
- Include lean protein and healthy fat in each snack and meal
- Choose vegetables and fruits that are rich in fiber
- Whenever possible choose organic and non-GMO foods

How Much:

- Small, frequent meals
- 3 meals with 2 snacks
- Appropriate portion sizes

Minimum per day:

- Include 1 legume as one of your daily protein grades
- Include 3-4 nuts/seeds as part of your daily fat grades
- Include 4 veggies per day

When: Start the day with breakfast and eat approximately every 3 hours after that

How:

- Enjoy your food and eat slowly
- Relax, eat with awareness – eat sensually!
- Enjoy your meals with friends and family

Chapter 5

Interstate Vixen12 – The Road Trip

Week 1

Get Your Inspection And Get Packed!

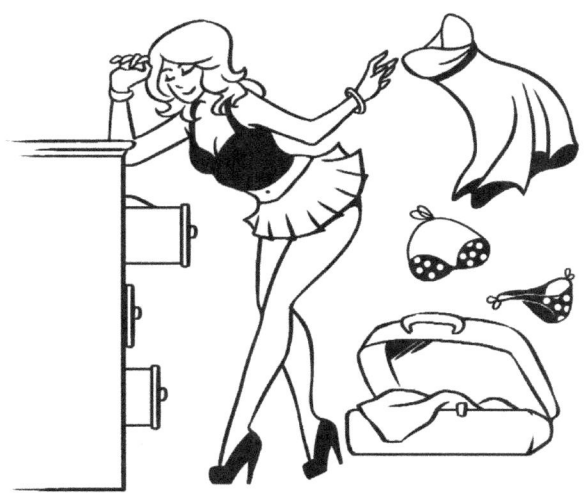

W hen I was growing up in North Carolina, once a year motorists had to take their car to a mechanic or quick lube joint to get inspected. Of course, the reason for this was to make sure that every car on the road was operating safely. Not all states require an inspection. But here, on Interstate Vixen12, we do. Your inspection for this road trip will be documenting your physical stats. When is the last time you got on the scale, measured your body fat, or took a hard look in the mirror?

As someone who has been where you are right now, I know that I used to avoid these things. I didn't want to know what

I weighed - if I could keep my head buried in the sand then I'd never have to DO anything about it. (Remember my overalls?) But closing your eyes to the truth causes you to be not fully present in your own life! The very first thing that you will do before getting in the car and driving off on Interstate Vixen12 to Freedom, is to take an honest assessment of where you are right now. This week you'll be learning about using metrics to track your success throughout the road trip. The two primary tools you'll be using will be the scale and the tape measure. These numbers will allow you to chart real measurable progress you are making, reinforce why exactly you are on this journey, and encourage you when you see those positive changes occurring. However, I also want to educate you on various methods of measuring body composition and body fat. More importantly, I want you to understand why using these tools can be beneficial in helping you gain optimal health to improve the quality of your life all around.

Women have a love-hate relationship with the scale. (For some of us, it may be more like hate-hate!) We see the number on the scale as a judge of our characters, thinking: *If I have a good number today, I am good. If I have a bad number today, I am bad.* You can substitute that word "bad" for "failure", "never going to get there", "wasting my time", or any other number of self-defeating words and phrases. But the scale is not your critic – it is simply a tool that gives you numerical feedback. I need you to address your fear of the scale right now, because you will become well acquainted with it over the next 12 weeks, and I hope for the rest of your life. If that scale does seem to be your critic, it is likely you are projecting your own criticism of yourself onto the scale. These are other issues we will be tackling throughout this program. So be patient, and remember that the mental, emotional and spiritual aspects of weight loss are equally as important as the physical ones. And your scale is used simply as a tool to help you stay on track.

Weighing yourself on a regular basis and using a scale consistently throughout life will prevent you from driving off course. If you wake up each day, or even once a week and step onto the scale — you will be able to spot those numbers creeping up before it gets out of your control. The real reason you avoid the scale might be because you can't handle the truth it is telling you. It is easy to convince yourself that the extra slice of cake didn't matter, when you don't have to see it reflected in the numbers on the scale. Keeping track will keep you honest and focused. It is much easier to make an immediate adjustment in diet or exercise to get the two pounds off that you gained, than it is to avoid the scale for five years and discover you have 60 lbs to lose. Trust me.

So if you do not have one, go out and purchase a scale. It may be helpful for you to weigh yourself daily, or maybe you are a once a week girl. If you like immediate feedback, and can view it is a tool and not character judge — daily may be the way for you to go. If you are someone who feels you need to see a good result, and cannot handle the stress of a daily weigh in — go for once a week. Regardless of when you perform this ritual, I want you to replicate the same circumstances each time. What you weigh naked first thing in the morning is not what you weigh at 6 PM with all of your clothes on. To get as accurate of a picture as possible — replicate the same circumstances every time. I strongly recommend that you weigh in first thing after waking, before eating or drinking, with no clothes on. Whatever method you choose, I want you to chart that number in your journal. Remember also, particularity for women, that hormones play a big roll in your weight. Eating salty foods, not drinking enough, over-drinking and eating excessive carbohydrates also factor into weight gain. If you weigh in daily, you may see fluctuations that make you unhappy, but as long as you see a decrease in weight overtime you are on the right track. If you "gain" two pounds in one day, it is safe to say that it is due to imbalances in your body and not actual weight gain. However, if after weighing yourself daily for three weeks, that two pounds is still there — it is probably fat. No matter what frequency and time you choose, I want you to begin to see the scale as a useful tool, and not your enemy.

The first step in your inspection process is taking your "before" picture. You can go crazy and take multiple shots in your underwear from various angles, or just a simple picture you take in the mirror is fine. Paste the photo on the front cover of your journal. However, if you think that the photo will inspire you daily if it is posted somewhere prominent, then by all means — tape it to the fridge or your bathroom mirror. Perhaps for you it will not be an encouragement and reminder of your goal, but will cause you to feel depressed or ashamed. If that is so, then own those feelings and keep your picture private in your journal for viewing when and where you choose. But know that it is not there as a means to punish you, but as a gentle reminder to urge you to keep pressing forward.

When tracking your success on any weight loss program, it can be very helpful to know your body composition and body fat, and there are several ways to gather this data. For example, many personal trainers use calipers to measure your Body Mass Index (BMI). There are also scales that you can purchase at practically any store that also calculate your BMI. If you want to go really high-tech then you can look into research labs that offer submersion techniques to determine your body mass and fat percentage. There is also something called bioelectrical impedance analysis (BIA), which electronically measures your body composition. Nothing will always be 100% accurate, but no matter which method you choose to use, if you continually use the same tool to measure yourself, you can at least chart the change. Muscle weighs more than fat, and as you get stronger your body composition will change when fat is replaced with lean tissue. So, keep this in mind if you see your pants-size dropping, but the number on your scale remains the same. If you feel good, have more energy and your clothing is getting looser, then no matter what the metrics show, you are doing something right.

Throughout this trip you will be changing your body composition, and that will be better reflected in inches lost and clothing sizes, than it will be in your weight. So in the next step of your inspection process, you'll be measuring your current "inches" and to do this, you will need a flexible tape measure. After taking these measurements, record them in your journal. You will be taking five measurements and doing a little easy math. You may want to take them more than once just to double-check yourself. Complete this in a full-length mirror so that you can ensure that you are holding the tape taught and level.

Chest: Measure around the fullest part of your bust wearing a bra that you will wear for every measurement. Be sure that the tape measure is level all the way around. Pull the tape taught and snug, it should not be drooping or loose, nor so tight it digs in.

Biceps: Measure your bicep midway between the shoulder and the elbow.

Waist: The World Health Organization recommends that you measure the area between the top of your hip or iliac crest and bottom of your lowest rib. For women your waist circumference should be less than 35 inches (32 inches for Asian women) and less than 40 inches for men (less than 35 inches for Asian men). If not, you are at a higher risk for obesity related illnesses. [5]

Hips: Stand with heels together and measure your hips across the widest part of your backside. Now calculate your waist to hip ratio

---

5 Waist circumference and waist–hip ratio: report of a WHO expert consultation, Geneva, 8–11 December 2008. http://whqlibdoc.who.int/publications/2011/9789241501491_eng.pdf

(WHR) by dividing your waist circumference by the circumference of your hips. Ratio for women: less than .8. Ratio for men: less than 1.0. If your WHR is higher than .8 it puts you at a higher risk for metabolic syndrome and other obesity related complications. [6]

Thighs: Measure both thighs, since many people have one leg larger than the other. Stand with legs slightly apart and measure around the widest part of each thigh.

The last check for completing your inspection is simple: write down your clothing sizes. Of course, sizes vary; so take a closet survey and average your dress size, pants size, blouse size, underwear and bra sizes. Measurements and size changes will be the best feedback you receive that you are on the right track and losing weight consistently!

Fuel for the Journey

The next question to answer before you take off on Interstate Vixen 12 is how much fuel do you need to travel? The perfect answer is just enough to keep you alive and energized, while still losing weight. It is easier to tell you *what* to eat than it is to determine how much of it. Everybody is different – our age, hormones, size and activity level all play a role in how much we need to eat to lose. A more active or younger person can eat more and get the same results as an older or more sedentary person, but the two will require a different caloric intake per day.

---

6   Waist to Hip Ratio, Waist Circumference and BMI: What to use for Health Risk Indication and Why? Len Kravitz Ph.D. - http://www.drlenkravitz.com/Articles/waisttohip.html

So how do we calculate our calorie needs? First, you need to find out your basal metabolic rate (BMR). Your BMR is the minimum number of calories your body needs to survive, if you did nothing at all but lay around on the couch all day. Here is the formula for a woman to calculate her BMR: 655 + (4.35 x weight in pounds) + (4.7 x height in inches) - (4.7 x age in years) Try this formula with your own stats. The number you end up with is your BMR.

Once you've determined your BMR, then you'll use the Harris-Benedict formula. This is the standard formula used to calculate daily calories needed in order to maintain your body weight. To do this, you calculate your BMR by your daily activity level:

Sedentary – BMR x 1.2 – (work a desk job and getting little to no physical activity)

Somewhat Active – BMR x 1.375 – (exercise 1-3 times per week)

Active – BMR x 1.55 – (exercise 3-5 times per week)

Very Active – BMR x 1.725 – (exercise 6-7 times per week)

Extremely Active – BMR x 1.9 – (exercise every day plus have a very physical job or exercise twice per day)

The number you get here will be the number of calories you need to survive, based on your activity level. Be honest with your-self, and when in doubt – round down concerning your activity level. You have just determined your caloric needs to _maintain_ your body weight based on your activity level, if you make no changes in your diet or activity level at all. The next step is to find out how many calories you need to consume daily in order to _lose_ weight.

A pound of stored body fat contains approximately 3500 calories. If you create a deficit of 3500 calories per week (500/day), theo-retically you would lose 1 pound of fat per week. In order to lose 2 pounds of fat per week, you would want to create a deficit of 7000 calories per week (1000/day). A healthy goal is to lose no more than 1-2 pounds of fat per week. Therefore for ideal fat loss, you should strive to reduce your caloric intake by about 500 calories per day through a combination of diet *and* exercise. And, keep in mind that the American College of Sports Medicine recommends that women go no lower than 1200 calories per day.

Once you've determined your caloric needs to survive based on your BMR x your current activity level at that time, then subtract 500 from that number to get your daily caloric needs to LOSE FAT at a rate of 1 pound per week.

Here is an example:

Emily is 160 pounds. She's 5'6" (66 inches tall). She's 48 years old. She exercises 1-3 times/week. The formula: 655 + (weight x 4.35) + (height x 4.7) - (age x 4.7)

Emily's formula: 655 + (160 x 4.35) + (66 x 4.7) - (48 x 4.7)

Emily's BMR = 1436

Using the Harris – Benedict Equation[7] Emily's activity level is considered somewhat active, so we multiply her BMR (1,436) by her activity level (1.375) and we come up with her caloric needs to maintain her body weight. 1,436 x 1.375 = 1,975 (rounded) In order to calculate a loss of 1 pound of fat per week, we would subtract 500 calories from 1,975. So Emily would need to consume 1,475 calories daily to lose 1 pound of fat per week. Emily's daily caloric goal: 1200-1475 calories, in order to lose 1-2 pounds/fat per week.

Once you determine the range of calories needed to lose 1-2 pounds of fat per week, use the chart in Chapter 4, the *High Octane Diet* to

---

7   J. Arthur Harris and Francis G. Benedict. Washington, DC: Carnegie Institution, 1919.

determine how many grades of each food group you will need to consume daily, in order to reach your caloric goals. You'll also want to track your food grades and ensure that you are weighing and measuring your food accurately. You can track your daily eating habits by simply creating a tally. On a page in your journal, make a list of your food categories, "protein", "fat", "veggie", "fruit", "starch", "dairy". Then, for example: if you require 11 protein grades per day, beside the word, "protein" you can put a slash mark every time you eat a grade of protein until you've reached 11. Then of course, you would do the same for the other food categories. Start a new page for each day. However, if you would prefer a tracking tool to help you with this, go to: www.vixenunleashed.com

As you lose weight, and as you increase your activity level, your maintenance number will CHANGE! You will need to account for this change as you lose the weight. So, periodically go back and do your calculations again, based on your new weight and activity level. Whatever you do, don't get discouraged because it might take you a little longer than expected. This isn't a sprint to the finish line; this is your journey and it will take practice and patience. The weight didn't get there overnight, nor will it leave you overnight. And if you're tired of yo-yo dieting, and you want long-term results, remember that making changes a little at a time is how you will do it. And if you apply those small changes *consistently,* over time you will achieve exactly what you're looking for, and more!

> Small Changes
> + Consistency
> = Success.

Pump up the tires

Your weight loss will come faster once you begin a solid exercise program, and your heart, lungs, and family will thank you as well.

But trust me — this is going to be a process. I don't want you to go hit the treadmill for 2 hours until you feel like your legs will fall off! Your exercise program will develop slowly over the next several weeks. My goal is to help you incorporate exercise into your life so you can make it a lifelong habit to be truly enjoyed. BUT, for now, your instructions are simple: if you are already exercising on a regular basis, keep doing it. If you are not, I recommend exercising two times per week, for a total of thirty minutes each time. It doesn't really matter what form of exercise you choose. The important thing is to commit to exercise of some sorts to get your heart rate elevated and your muscles moving. You could power walk with a friend, watch a fitness DVD, join a gym, swim or take up dancing. One friend of mine lost 25 pounds just doing one of those dance video games with her kids! (This is an excellent way to bond with your kids and lose some weight too!) On two of the days that you're not doing your 30 minutes/ 2 x week… I'd like for you to go outside and take a casual walk and get some fresh air… and either listen to upbeat, positive music or affirmations on your MP3 player, or say affirmations to yourself while you walk. This will help make the mind/body connection and uplift your spirit. I created a great affirmation CD that I used as I was going through my personal weight loss journey. You can find that at: www.vixenunleashed.com .

GET YOUR MOTOR RUNNING

Are you ready to start supercharging your body? I'm going to let you in on an energy-boosting secret! I call it, "V12 Turbo-Boost".

This 12-minute addition to your exercise regime is based off of a fat blasting concept called High Intensity Interval Training. It involves pushing up your intensity level for short bursts of time, followed by a period of rest. It is VERY important that before beginning the V12 Turbo-Boost exercises, that you consult with your doctor and make sure that your health can handle High Intensity Interval Training. If you are totally sedentary, and out of shape, or haven't exercised for a long time, then I want you to ease into this and wait until you've built up your other exercises, lost some weight, and are feeling stronger. When you're feeling ready, and your doctor gives you the "go ahead," then you can start the V12 Turbo-Boost for a total of 12 minutes per session, five days per week. You can do it when it is convenient for you, but I recommend first thing in the morning if you can. It is also a great tool to use in the afternoon when you may crave that energy boost you get from a soda or sugary snack. I used to grab 12 minutes on a short break while I was at work each afternoon, by using a step stool I had in my office! Your V12 Turbo-Boost can be done with any high intensity exercise you like – running, stair climbing, jumping jacks, or squats. Walking for your low intensity time, with sprints for your high intensity time is probably the easiest form of High Intensity Interval Training to do. So, for my example we'll use walking and sprinting:

It's simple – imagine a scale of 1-10, 1 being the least amount of effort, 10 being maximum effort or intensity. (Keep in mind that your highest intensity may be different than someone else's.) You'll start by warming up at a gentle walking pace for 1 minute. Then, for 30 seconds you will sprint at the intensity of your "8-9", and then drop back to an intensity of "2" and walk for 3 minutes. Repeat this sequence until you have reached 12 minutes. That's it.

The benefits of exercise go much deeper than fat loss or increased lung and heart capacity. The endorphins released through exercise will make you feel good in the moment and after the work is complete. The self esteem you derive from accomplishing your physical goals — whether it be to ride the bike longer or walk faster, will increase your sense of self worth and personal power in all areas of life. The mental benefit includes relaxation, stress and anxiety relief and an ability to solve problems. Great thoughts and ideas can come to you when your body is occupied in physical activity and your mind is free to wander and ponder. Exercise in this context cannot be seen as a chore, but as a way to put yourself first, to kindly take care of your whole woman — mind, body and spirit. I want you to forget what you know about exercise and try to get a hold on this concept — if you can find something that you love to participate in; it will not feel like a drudge — but a joy!

You will be doing the aforementioned exercise routine for the next 4 weeks. Each month we will be building upon your exercise routine, and your instructions for that change will be found in your action steps at Mile Markers 1, 5 and 9. But don't panic, I want you to stay focused on one week at a time. Right now — for the first month you will be doing something 5 days per week. But it's not a crazy amount. Think about it… really, you're only doing 30 minutes of exercises, two times per week and taking a casual walk twice per week, choosing the pace that YOU want. And, if the doc says you can, then you're doing five weekly sessions of V12 Turbo-Boost, each being ONLY 12 minutes long. That's it! If possible, I do recommend doing your V12 Turbo Boost the first thing in the morning… to get your blood moving, energy level up and start boosting your metabolism right away!

I've presented you with a lot of information designed to get your car ready to travel. In the next week you'll take a Road Test to help you assess your mindset and emotions, and help you to discover your inner Vixen. The answer to those questions will guide you in knowing your dream and setting your goals, as well as determine what your road-blocks could be on this trip. We've kicked the tires and given the car a once over, but in the following pages we're going to look under the hood and find out why you've really put yourself in the back seat instead of the driver's seat. Hold on to your hats gals, we're going for a ride!

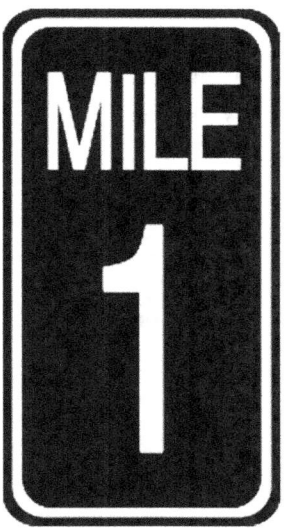

ACTION STEPS

- Weigh and measure yourself, record your sizes and test your hip-waist ratio. Take a "before" photo of yourself. Record all of this data on the front pages of your journal.
- Keep track of every meal you eat and the time you eat them in a journal. Keep the journal with you so you don't forget anything.
- Using the formulas given, calculate your BMR, multiply it by your activity level, and then subtract 500 from it to determine

your daily caloric intake to lose fat. Reference the chart in the *High Octane Diet* to determine how many grades of each food source you need daily. Track your grades in your journal, or use the resources at: www.vixenunleashed.com .

- Eliminate all refined sugars, wheat and gluten from your diet. Choose foods from the food list in the *High Octane Diet*. For a 14-day sample diet, go to: www.vixenunleashed.com.
- Focus on eating 5-6 small meals per day, including protein in each meal and try to space your meals out approximately every 3 hours.
- Complete a 12 minute V12 Turbo-Boost session, once per day for five days, and choose some sort of exercise to do for 30 minutes, 2 x per week.
- Take 2 casual walks per week, listening to positive music or affirmations while you walk.
- Weigh in daily or weekly and track your changes.
- Drink 8-10 cups of water each day

Week 2

Where Are You Right Now?

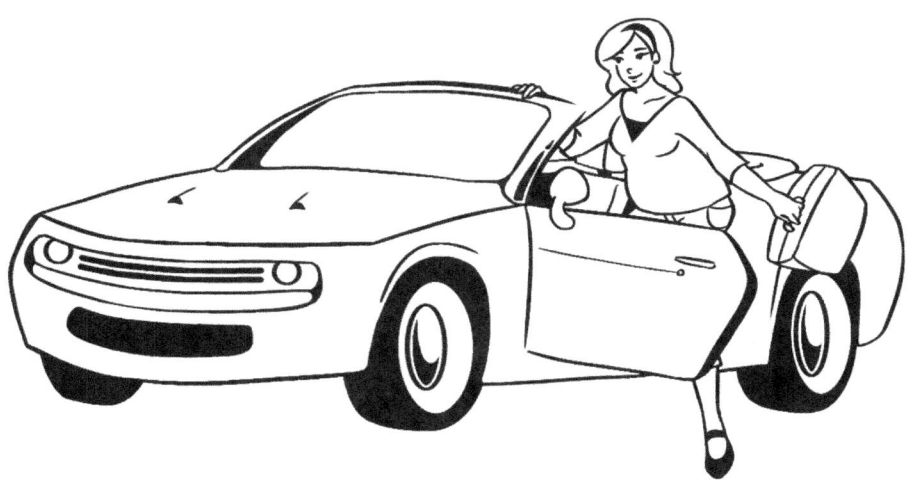

N ow that you know the foundation of your diet and exercise plan, we're almost ready to go! But first, it's time for your Road Tests. If you want to get the most out of these 12 weeks, you absolutely won't want to "cheat" on your road tests... These two quizzes will serve as the foundation of all the changes you desire to make. To truly unleash your inner Vixen, you have to know more than just an eating and exercise plan, you have to become deeply acquainted with yourself. And that's what this next week is all about. In this coming week we will be tackling some heavy issues that may make you uncomfortable. For some women, it can be much easier to deal with outer fat than inner pain. But to completely transform, the change must begin on the inside. So grab your map and let's go on a journey…inside of you.

You will be taking 2 tests that will reveal some of your deepest thoughts and feelings, as well as pinpointing your core values. These tests will allow you to understand what roadblocks you might encounter and help you set goals based on who you are as a woman. In addition, this week you will spend some quality time in the mirror learning to love yourself, and I'll show you how gratitude plays an important role in developing the new attitude you need to be a strong and sensual vixen.

If you remember, I didn't feel too sexy when I went to my first pole dancing class. When the class began, I had difficulty lifting my heavy body up the pole. So the instructor loaned me a pair of knee-high vinyl boots to give me a little extra grip. While I was dancing around the pole, I watched my reflection in the mirror and interestingly, I found myself staring at my legs; in awe of the way those boots showcased how long they were. This was quite strange for me, because normally I would have been focusing on my huge, dimpled thighs. That incident spawned a decision to begin consciously looking for positive attributes in myself every time I looked in the mirror, with the goal of letting go of my negative self-image. And little by little my practice paid off. So when developing this program, I used this practice to create a few simple daily exercises that will help you to narrow in on the good qualities you have, and move away from any habits of being critical of yourself.

ROAD TESTS

The first test you'll be taking is the Introspection Quiz (your IQ test). It was designed to help you understand who you really are, what motivates you, and how you see yourself. By knowing your authentic self; the person you really are deep within, you will lay a foundation that will ultimately help you break through frustrations, end bad habits, change your attitude towards food and exercise, find your inner sexy, and lose your outer fat. The more clear that you are about who you are; the easier it will be for you to reach your goals and create the body you desire and life that you deserve. Please keep in mind that I've been down this path myself, and I know the emotional pain and discomfort associated with facing truths. It isn't easy, and still even today I have to refer back to my road tests to help me get back on track in life when I notice things starting to get out of balance. And remember, this evaluation is for you to get real with yourself, and you are the only one that will see this. If you've never been totally honest with yourself and have been burying your head in the sand about your emotions and your body, now is time to open your eyes. This is an opportunity for you to take inventory of where you are now, to pinpoint your strengths and weaknesses, and to uncover the truth. Don't feel any shame or embarrassment; many women have struggled with weight problems, self-esteem issues, and emotional eating as well. As a matter of fact, studies have shown that 97% of women had at least one negative thought about their body daily. [8]So, you are not alone in this process, I assure you.

As you go through this IQ test, be prepared to uncover what you might consider to be imperfections and weaknesses. Within those weaknesses and imperfections you will discover a beauty and a strength that is more incredible than you can imagine. Find a time to do this when you can sit down by yourself and focus in, without interruption, and get real. This may take an hour or so, depending on

---

8 March 2012 issue Glamour Magazine http://www.glamour.com/health-fitness/2011/02/shocking-body-image-news-97-percent-of-women-will-be-cruel-to-their-bodies-today

how deep you are willing to dig. If you need to take a break at any point and go back to it later, please do.

Make sure that you really think about the questions, and answer them honestly. Don't simply put down what you think is correct or appropriate! Do not be ashamed of your answers or feelings — they are yours, and you must own them! You should be proud of yourself for taking this HUGE step. It's like turning the key in the ignition - it has to be done before the car can go forward. Without doing this first, you'll never be able to drive to your destination. Don't worry about what you see in the rearview mirror as you go through this assessment. It is a reminder of why you are driving into a new life. You'll find the "IQ" test in the back of this book. Please use your journal to write down the answers.

CORE VALUES

Your next test is called your Core Values Test. Before you journey on down Interstate Vixen 12, you're going to be taking some time to identify what is deeply important to you. Your core values are often not a choice; they are part of who you innately are. Knowing these truths about yourself will help you to pinpoint what will motivate you to unleash your inner Vixen, drop the weight and reach Freedom.

More importantly, this knowing will help you to fully love your-self and embrace life with passion and joy.

In the core values test you will answer a series of questions about qualities you honor in others and find in yourself to be most authentically "you". In the final test you will select words from a list that draw your attention. Try not to over-think the words on this list. Often we want to describe ourselves in a certain way, such as "kind" or "spiritual" or "competent", but in actuality the words or concepts that pull us might be "freedom", "adventure" and "courage". You may also be kind and competent, but these are secondary traits and ones that you spend time cultivating. Who you are deeply will call to you; answer the call! As with all the work you're doing in this program, be sure to write down your answers to these questions in your journal.

It is important that you own these core value traits, and accept them. Perhaps they are not what you want them to be, but they are you - so you should embrace them and be proud! All of these values, whether you have been aware of it or not, are a major driving force behind every decision you make. For example, if your top core value is "acceptance", many of the actions you take on a daily basis have been structured to gain the acceptance you seek. Maybe this results in you being a people pleaser, and perhaps when you let people down or are in conflict, you are driven to overeat to handle those feelings of rejection. The goal isn't to change your core values, but to celebrate them and understand a new way of using them to your advantage instead. In this case, for example, you might want to take that core value and strive for self-acceptance rather than always striving for acceptance from others.

If you can remember and connect with your core values in everyday life, you will learn to make smart choices based upon them, choices that will intrinsically be pleasing to you. In addition, you should use your core values list to examine the people that you hang out with. Think this through carefully – are you spending time with people who support your core values? If you value your freedom but spend a lot of time with a friend who is bossy or controlling, this is not in support of your values and that relationship may be detrimental. Some relationships, such as those with close family, cannot be eliminated from our lives. In that circumstance, simply *knowing* that the reason your loved one can get under your skin is due to differing core values, can be extremely helpful in easing the tension! If punctuality is one of your core values, and your sister is late for everything, you will be better able to understand and forgive this action in her if you realize that deep in your core you are opposed to lateness. Punctuality is YOUR value, not hers. You are no more "right" than she is - just different! So go ahead, take a moment to reflect on the relationships you have. Is there anyone who doesn't support your core values? Are your relationships helpful or harmful? If you value your health, and a friend of yours drinks, smokes and goes out for daily happy hour appetizers – perhaps this relationship should be re-evaluated. Maybe you limit the amount of time you spend with that person or which activities you do with her. For friendships that are truly harmful, you may need to go so far as kicking people out of your life If you truly love the person in question and do not want to leave them behind, maybe the relationship needs to be marginalized a bit, or restructured. What if, instead of joining that friend at the bar on Tuesdays and Fridays, you start a book club and meet for tea once a week to talk about what you've read? If it has value to you, see if you can re-direct a relationship instead of just kicking it to the curb. If it is not worth salvaging a harmful relationship that is in opposition to your values, then you'll have to take action. Part of the journey to Freedom will involve tossing out baggage that is keeping you from reaching your full potential. And I can tell you from experience, that if you are feeling "stuck" and can't seem to create change that you desire, nine times out of ten its because of something or someone that you least expect, which is holding you back. And once you let go of that baggage, the energy begins to flow freely and results begin to manifest. Now, I'm not saying to go get a divorce or quit your job… because even though we might want to place blame on what seems to be the obvious, many times its something different. Its time to get introspective and real with yourself to see exactly what is holding you back from your dreams. This is a one-way journey, and some things will need to be left behind!

Knowing, thinking and embracing your core values EVERYDAY will enable you to make healthier, more positive choices, not only in your what you eat, but in everything you do. The first step to unleashing your inner Vixen is to unveil the real YOU, and to know what is truly valuable to you, deep inside. Once you experience that kind of self-knowing, your sensuality will begin to gently unfold, and your life will become richer. So, before reading on, go to the back of this book and take your IQ Test and your Core Values Test. Remember this when it comes to your truth and core values; your objection is simple:

> Find it.
> Own it.
> Live it.

USING YOUR MIRRORS
PART 1

As mentioned above, to truly set yourself free and unleash your inner Vixen, you will need to learn the discipline of self-love. The idea may even be ridiculous to you: *How could I love this mess? Have you seen my thighs, my rolls, and double chin? Please — maybe other women can do it. But I'M different, there is no way I could love this body! Not unless I lost 50 pounds first!*

That's a common thought, but I have news for you - if you are incapable of loving yourself, RIGHT NOW, just as you are — rolls and all, you will not be able to love yourself when you are thin. You will never be good enough. Your skin won't be as tight as you'd like, there will be a little bulge over here and there, you'll feel great in your clothes, but maybe not so much when unclothed. Truly loving yourself is not based on external circumstances, but on a change that you make within your heart. And this change starts simply: Step 1: Stop beating yourself up, Step 2: Re-focus.

Ok... so maybe it's not so simple. We are conditioned by years of external criticism from our parents, siblings, classmates, friends, media, and society to find all of the ways we fall short and don't fit in. When you look in the mirror or at a photo of yourself, where do your eyes always go? That's right – the part you hate the most! Is it your backside? Your stomach? Your thighs? Do you ever see your photo and think: *I have a great smile?* Or *Wow, look how nice my hair looked that day?* Probably not. Truly letting go of the negative focus takes a firm decision, discipline and consistency, and it is absolutely essential in your journey down Interstate Vixen12. No negativity is allowed! That negativity is baggage that you are going to take out of the trunk right now and toss out of the car! By the end of this journey I want to see you loving yourself the way others love you.

Would you look at your daughter or another little girl in your life, and say, "Ugh, you are so disgusting?" or "I hate your thighs, they look like tree trunks?" or "You can't put on a bathing suit, you are gross and everyone will laugh at you!" What was your gut reaction to those statements? Can you imagine looking an innocent, tenderhearted little girl in the face and unleashing such criticism on her spirit? NEVER! You wouldn't dream of doing such a thing to an impressionable child! So, what gives you the right to do it to yourself? It is your job to protect and nurture your heart first, so why do you constantly speak those vile words to yourself? Research tells us that the thoughts and words we repeat over and over seep into

our subconscious and come to define us. For years you've probably been defining yourself as "failure" or "slob" or "ugly" or "unworthy". How can you expect that you'd feel sexy? How could you ever
reach Freedom, and be the woman you always hoped you'd be, if on
every moment of the journey you've got this critic in the passenger's
seat telling you that you are a pig and you'll always be fat, and not
to bother? You couldn't! And my friend, that critic, the one who is
always with you and dishes it out mercilessly - is you. There will
always be negative outside influences, but every one of them can be
combated by a serious commitment to self-love.

So, what can be done? First, I want you to work on eliminating
the negativity. When you go clothes shopping look at photo albums
or stare in the mirror – you will not utter the words, back fat, cankles
or bat wings. In fact, go ahead and ban those words right now from
your vocabulary! They are not funny – they are hurtful. Next, keep
a mini notebook and pencil with you at all times this entire week.
Every time you catch yourself thinking a negative thought or saying
something negative or hurtful about your body, reach into your purse
and write down the exact words you just thought or said. At the end
of the day, you'll be shocked at how hard you are on yourself. Then,
I want you to rip those pages out of the notebook, crumple them up
and throw them in the trash… or better yet, burn them! This will
get you in the habit of recognizing how much you punish yourself,
to help prevent you from doing it repeatedly. The act of throwing
those words away will help your subconscious start to believe that
you don't want those negative self-image words in your life!

The next step in this process is equally as important – to begin
identifying things about yourself, outer and inner qualities, that you
like and appreciate, and reinforce those positive thoughts consistently
and often. I want you to stand in front of a mirror at least one time
each day and have an honest look. Try hard to find something nice to

say about you, preferably out loud. This may be very hard at first and you'll have to dig deep, but there is SOMETHING you like physically, I am sure of it. Perhaps it's your height, your hair color, your eyes or freckles. Perhaps you have a nice chest, or you have nice curves. Tell yourself this truth lovingly, and believe it. Repeat it to yourself again and again. Remember earlier when I told you that research has shown how repeated thoughts and words sink into our subconscious and come to define us? This is why repeating *positive* thoughts and words over and over is so important! It works both ways. After years of negative conditioning, its time to re-condition your mind. You'll feel silly at first, but that's okay. You may want to put a note on your bathroom mirror that says "Remember: Positivity!" or "Love yourself today!" as a reminder to practice this discipline. And that is what it is – a discipline. At first this may feel forced and inauthentic, but with time you will come to really believe these statements about yourself, I promise.

In addition, I want you to be thinking inwardly during this mirror exercise. Tell yourself what it is you like about your personality. When all else fails, and you are having a miserable no good day and just cannot bring yourself to say anything nice about your body, then double your focus on your inner woman, and tell her how wonderful she is! That you appreciate her kindness, or that she is a good mother, or that she is a hard worker. You will have to practice being patient and kind with yourself as you learn to do this. Stay consistent, and you will experience genuine change about how you feel about your body, and it will even translate over into how you view the world. When you begin to shift your gaze from negative personal thoughts to positive ones, it will carry over into other areas of your life, including your relationships.

THE GRATITUDE WHEEL
PART 1

That thought leads us to the final discipline in this week: gratitude. Think of the Gratitude Wheel as your steering wheel on the road to Freedom. If you grasp gratitude firmly with both hands, someone can come along and blindside you, but your car will stay firmly on the right path. Just like a steering wheel, the Gratitude Wheel is divided into three sections. We will address the first section during this week. You'll learn about Part 2 and Part 3 of the Gratitude Wheel as we travel down Interstate Vixen12.

Are you grateful for what you have right now in life? Or are you spending your time thinking about what you want but don't have – a thinner body, more money, a better job, a happier relationship? When things get stressful or life gets challenging, if you were to take a few moments to focus on one particular thing that you are truly grateful for – your whole outlook could change! If you practice this discipline everyday, it could change you permanently; you could change from a negative person, to a positive one, from someone who sweats the small stuff to someone who's oblivious to it, from someone who is a victim in life to a victor!

There is always something to be grateful for! Think about it – instead of complaining about rush hour traffic, try being grateful that you had a car to sit in and a job to go to! Instead of complaining how hot it is outside, why not look around and be thankful for the lovely green trees and flowers that you enjoy seeing in the summer. Instead of complaining about how your husband doesn't understand you, be grateful that you were able to find a partner who loves you and to enjoy life with.

One great trick that I used during my own weight loss journey was to spend some time each day practicing gratitude. Being grateful for what you have now is the first discipline of the Gratitude Wheel. Each morning upon waking, I opened my journal, and wrote down three things that I was grateful for. I tried not to write the same three things everyday, but some days I did. Sometimes it was the weather, material possessions, relationships, or health, whatever came to me in that moment. Then I would sit and ponder each thing I named. I would repeat each one to myself again and again until I could actually begin to *feel* and experience real gratitude, saying, "I am so grateful that I have my son" or "I am so grateful that my parents are around for me to spend time with". During that daily exercise, I would commit those three items to memory, and throughout my day I would speak them to myself again. I want you to implement this practice at a time when it is convenient for you to complete during the day. Morning is a great time, because it sets the tone for the whole day, but you can practice it in the evening as you reflect on your day as well.

All of us have relationship troubles at one time or another with friends, siblings, parents, co-workers or our spouse. Using gratitude is a wonderful way to thwart relationship woes in particular, and stop you from medicating your negative feelings with food. If you are having an argument with your husband, and he is throwing darts at you — instead of throwing them back, you can make the conscious choice to think in your heart about what you really love and value in him (even if you can't see it right now!). It'll change your demeanor, tone, and feelings. You will work from a place of acceptance and thankfulness and not be participating in tearing down that relationship; instead you'll be working on building it up.

These mantras created a daily change in me - to refocus on what I love, what was valuable, and to stop sweating the small stuff. It is easy to think about everything that is wrong, but on Interstate Vixen12 we are going to learn to think about everything that is right instead! Truly – a grateful attitude is the foundation of an unshakable life, that won't be rattled by minor annoyances or even large problems. It will keep you focused and steering strongly on the straight and narrow towards a life you always dreamed of. Being grateful and expressing it is so important on this journey – you must not skip this discipline. Trust me, the work is worth it!

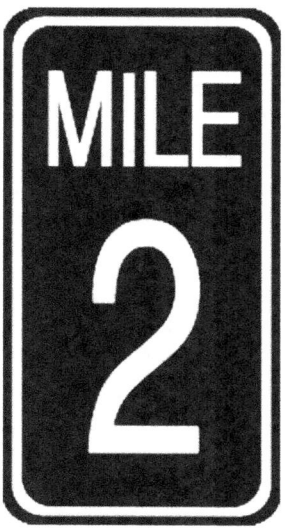

ACTION STEPS

- Complete the Road Test and the Core Values Test located in the back of the book
- Record in a notebook your daily negative self-image thoughts and words. At night, crumple up the paper that they're written on and throw it in the trash!

- Start practicing self-love by naming your positive attributes in the mirror daily
- Implement the first discipline of the Gratitude Wheel by meditating on what you are thankful for each day
- Continue with the *High Octane Diet*
- Continue with your workout regime
- Weigh in daily or weekly and track your changes.
- Drink 8-10 cups of water each day

Week 3

Where Are You Going?

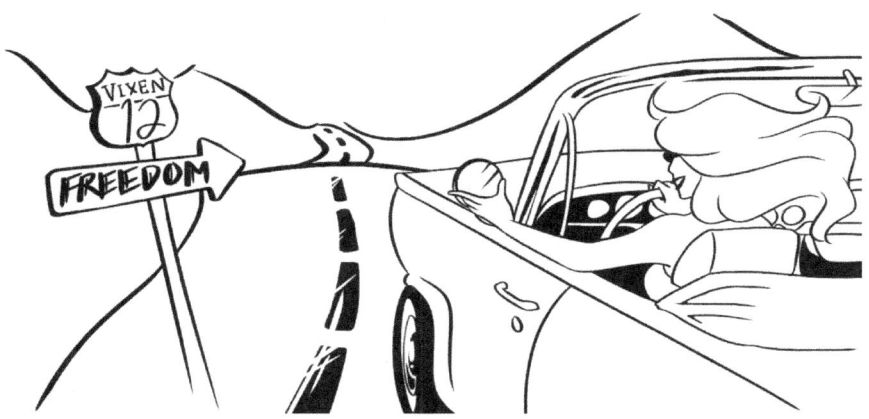

L ast week you spent time getting real with yourself and learning about what you value most. Now that you have a better grasp of what is truly important to you, you are going to create a vision of who you want to be and what the town of Freedom looks like for YOU! During this week you will be learning skills that will change your outlook and self-perception. Once you have created a clear vision of the woman you want to be, you will be able to map out the steps needed to bring that Vixen to life. Remember how I told you that these small changes you make would eventually lead to your greater vision? It's true! And a very important component to this 12-week program is that you continue to practice the exercises from the previous weeks, while adding in these new disciplines. This week you will be creating a travel-sized Vixen Vision board, that will allow you to put into words and images exactly who you aspire to be. You will set your GPS coordinates for your ultimate destination – the town of Freedom, where the happy, healthy, sexy you resides, and you will learn more about how gratitude can shape your route on Interstate Vixen12, and how it can change your life.

When I was plotting my course to Freedom, I thought it would help to make a Vision Board. I could always use it as encouragement and inspiration along the way, and remind myself of why I was making these new healthy choices and changing my attitude. I filled it with phrases and pictures that represented the woman I wanted to become. It was a strong reflection of my core values. As my number one value is "freedom", it was no surprise that my Vision board was populated with images and words relating to that concept. On the center of my board I placed the most important picture – a photo that best represented to me, the feelings of "freedom". It represented my inner Vixen. It was a photo showing a woman, standing in the rain, in a forest of vibrant green trees. In the picture, even though it was raining… there were rays of sunshine filtering through the leaf cover. Her face was turned upward to the brightening sky. She looked elated and serene and utterly unburdened, just like I imagined freedom to be! My Vision Board allowed me to visually express my hopes and dreams for myself, and you will be making a similar board to help you to define where you are going, and as a reminder of who you're becoming.

Travel sized Vixen vision board
Part 1

Creating your Vixen vision board allows you to develop a visual picture of the woman you want to transform into, on the inside and out. Your board will actually be small and portable. It will be your personal travel brochure that you can carry with you on your journey, and refer to often so you can remain focused on your goal. So get out your glue and scissors - it's time for an art project! (Don't worry if you aren't crafty – anyone can do this assignment!) This exercise will help you project those core values onto something productive, and result in a tangible object you can use to reaffirm why you are doing this for yourself.

For your travel brochure, you will need a piece of 8.5 X 11 card stock or poster board, which you will fold in thirds, like a business letter (not accordion style, but folding the outer edges in). On the front cover, write "My Vixen Vision", and there you will glue a photo of the outer Vixen you plan to become physically. This can be an old photo of you, in days when you were happy, healthy and fit, or it can be a picture ripped from a magazine, catalog or one you pulled from the web. Wherever you get it, do your best to make sure it is realistic. If you are 5'11" tall and have a large bust, don't choose a picture of a petite, small-breasted woman – that is unreasonable. You should stretch and dream big, but accept that there are genetic components that no amount of diet, exercise and determination can change!

Opening the brochure up will reveal three inside panels. In the center panel, you will attach or draw another picture. This picture is representative of the woman you envision yourself to be on the inside (like my picture of "freedom"). This can be simple or elaborate – it's your board, so you decide. You can draw a smiley face, find stock photos on the web, or cut pictures out of a magazine. Perhaps what you want most is to feel serene and peaceful inside — and maybe an image of the ocean at sunset evokes that particular feeling in you. Is adventure you highest core value? Then maybe a photo of a rock climber hanging over a canyon creates that sense of danger and adrenaline you want to achieve. Choose a picture that emulates what you dream to feel.

The next step in designing your travel-size Vixen Vision board is decorating the inside left panel — here you will be writing simple, one word descriptors of the woman you will be physically. Take a few moments to daydream about her- is she muscular, voluptuous, flexible? Is she curvy or lean? Is she strong, thin, and energetic? You can use these words, but I encourage you to spend time imagining her appearance and coming up with your own words for your board. You may want to write her measurements or her dress size or describe the type of clothes she wears. Begin to envision yourself completely as her; put your face on that body you see in your mind — it is you!

Finally, for your descriptive words on the right hand panel you will follow the same exercise, only using your inner self as the inspiration. Who is that inner Vixen? How do you feel as you unleash her; what will you love and value? Do you feel freedom or lightness? Are you centered or in balance for the first time? Do you have pride in yourself for once? Truly envision those inner feelings and emotions, and describe your spirit!

Now that you have filled in the "what" of your future, in coming weeks you will also be filling in the "why". For now, just keep your focus on the inner panels; they are a great start towards steering your thinking in the right direction.

SET YOUR DESTINATION

Before going on a trip to a place you've never been, you most likely pull out your GPS device and punch in the address or coordinates of where you are headed. If you don't, you'd be driving aimlessly — with nothing but hope that you'll end up in the right spot. However, if you set those coordinates and follow the directions exactly, you WILL get to where you hoped to go. It is the same way on this road trip — if you set your coordinates, and plot your path, you simply have to stay on Interstate Vixen12 until you reach your destination!

I have a friend who has one of those fussy European cars, and a computer controls all of the car's mechanical functions. If the tiniest thing goes wrong, such as when she forgets to tighten the gas cap down, it activates a sensor, which causes a warning light to go on. But even after she remedies the situation, by re-tightening the gas cap, the "check engine" light stays on! The only way to turn the warning light off is to take it to the shop and spend $20 to have the computer reset, a task she has to do more frequently than she'd like. I find this interesting - she doesn't simply need to remove the problem, she needs to take ACTION to reset the brain of the car. Similarly — you are removing negativity, but you still need to take action to replace it with something better. This week, you are going to do just that, by learning how to reprogram your subconscious thinking!

How can you reprogram your brain and change the way you have always viewed yourself? It sounds difficult, but it is actually very doable. Let me explain - the negative thoughts you often have are what scientists refer to as "automatic thoughts", knee-jerk subconscious responses to particular stimuli (in this case, your view of yourself). For example - every time you get undressed in the bathroom mirror, you may think the same cruel words about your body. Or each time you think about losing weight you have the same defeatist attitude. If you habitually do this, you are practically destined to fail. You are blocking your own success and placing undesirable limitations on yourself due to your belief system. It is not what you say or even think about yourself that is the problem, but what you *believe about yourself*. Research suggests that the only way to change these automatic thoughts is to change your *beliefs,* using Cognitive Behavior Therapy (CBT). Instead of believing that you are destined to fail, you will reprogram yourself to believe you can't fail. Instead of believing that it is okay to say cruel words about your body, because you aren't worth much anyway, you'll learn that you are valuable and worthy of love and respect. When you accept that as true, your knee jerk reaction will not be to put yourself down. Your automatic responses will reflect this new belief. You will begin replacing those "I can't" thoughts with "I will" thoughts and words! And once you begin to think and speak like a successful person, you will be actively changing your thought patterns. CBT is best performed under the guidance of a therapist if you have deeper anxiety, anger or other emotional issues. However, for our purposes here, you can successfully use some of these principals to change your beliefs about yourself.

Before beginning this exercise, take a few moments to reflect on your core values. All of your future goals should be based around the words you identified with. In your journal, you will be creating three GPS pages, labeled "Mind", "Body", and "Spirit". On these pages you will write down your specific goals in these three areas of your life. There is one special instruction – you must write everything in the present tense! This is how you will program your GPS, and begin changing your beliefs about yourself. Yes, these are goals that you have not achieved…YET. But if you can capture an image of yourself this way – if you can believe that you innately are this woman, then that is what you will become. This journey to Freedom really starts with you convincing yourself you already are FREE!

On the page you have labeled "Body", write out your goals as if you have attained them. Use statements such as: "I have lost 20 pounds", "I am a size 8", "I run four days per week", "I climb mountains each weekend", etc. These should be specific descriptive statements about your physical state and the life you are able to live with your new sexy and healthy body. On the page that is labeled "Mind" you will list goals you have for your mental and emotional state, using statements like "I am content with my life", "I have a sense of freedom", "I feel at peace and in control", etc. Remember to refer to your core values to help you set these goals! For example, if "security" was one of your values, then you may want to make one of your goals, "I feel secure".

The third page of your GPS, "Spirit" will be just as individual to you as your mind and body pages are. Are you a religious person or do you label yourself as "spiritual'…or are you neither? I believe, no matter what you want to call it – God, the Universe, or something else – there is a Higher Power in each of us… our Higher Self. The benevolent, caring and peaceful side of your person should be nurtured and grown during this journey as well. What good is a gorgeous body, with a deadened spirit?

I personally know a beautiful, fit woman, who exercises regularly and eats a clean, healthy diet, but she allows stress to consume her. She is constantly complaining about her "to-do" list with not enough time in the day to complete everything needed to be done; so she's running around like a mad woman all the time. She desperately wants somebody to help her, because she feels like she's alone. However, she also feels like nobody can do things as well as she can, so she has to take control, and do everything herself. Where is the problem here? She eats right, exercises, and takes care of her body…but she is lacking in taking care of her spirit. Here is the thing…. YES, a schedule is good! If you are a busy woman, in order to accomplish everything you want in a day, you have to have a schedule that you go by, which will give you a certain amount of control (we talk about the importance of schedules later in the program). But in order to have *sanity* in your life, reduce the stress, and give you a more balanced and harmonious life, you also need to relinquish control. It's somewhat of an oxymoron. You need to recognize that you are not separate from the Universe… you are NOT alone… and you are part of a greater energy. And when you deeply connect with your Divine Feminine… with your spirit energy… you will realize that in order to have control, you must release control. By that, I mean to trust that the Universe has your back… and everything WILL be okay. It may not always work out the way you think it should…but it WILL be okay, and it will be good… if you just trust, let go, and let God. If my friend would only nurture her spirit woman, she would discover that everything she was worried about wasn't really a worry at all. She has so many wonderful things going on for her, but what is missing is her willingness to be introspective, connect with her soul and honor her spirit.

As you can see by this example, goals for your spirit woman are equally important in this trio of mind, body, and spirit, if you seek to create a better version of YOU. So think about your spirit goals and write them out. They can be anything from "I attend church regularly" to " I meditate daily" or, "I trust in my higher-power and every day I practice letting go of the need to control". Remember, this is YOUR spirit goal and should reflect your personal spiritual beliefs. Nurturing this part of yourself will create balance in your life, peace and gratitude in your interactions, respect and mindfulness for yourself and the rest of society. Everyone needs to quiet down, unplug from the demands of life, and seek the sacred. Make it your goal to find a way to gain peace and access the Higher Power within you. Use descriptive actions about how you are nourishing your spirit.

You are working to change your view of yourself; this is a practice that needs to be done consistently. So, now that you have written out specific goals for mind, body and spirit, and learned how to speak about those results as if you've already attained them, let's go back to the mirror and see how you can change your views while gazing at your reflection.

USING YOUR MIRRORS
PART 2

Last week you learned how to use the mirror to see your positive traits, now I want you to learn the skill of using the mirror to visualize the woman you are becoming; your future YOU. Each day you will spend a few moments staring at your reflection, verbalizing the awesomeness of your body, as if you had already reached your "body" goals. Complete this the same way you did your GPS work - in the present tense: "I love my new, slender body", "My thighs are gorgeous, lean and strong", "I look incredible in my size 6 jeans", etc. Do this in the morning, after you have done your morning gratitude exercise. You will already be in a state of thankfulness, and it will be easier to connect with those positive feelings about the woman you'll become. You may feel silly doing this, or like you are lying to yourself, but you aren't — you are simply seeing your future body right now! This exercise is designed to feed your subconscious mind new truths about yourself, and if you practice this regularly your body cannot help but follow. Remember, in order to change your feelings about yourself, you have to change your beliefs. Believe you are capable of success by reinforcing this truth.

~~~~~~~~~~

THE GRATITUDE WHEEL
PART 2

In addition to your "future you" mirror exercises, you will also take time to express thanks for your desired Vixen in your journal each night. This is part 2 of the Gratitude Wheel - learning how to be grateful for what you don't have...yet! Through this discipline you will be teaching your subconscious mind that what you dream yourself to be one day, already exists now. The more you work on this, the quicker your mind will believe it and the faster your body will change.

Every night before bed, take a few moments to write down in your journal three things that you are most grateful for, as if you have already reached your goal. It is important that you choose one goal from each of your three GPS pages. Express your gratitude for your achievements in mind, body and spirit using present tense statements. One day's entry might read: "I am grateful that I have lost 18 inches", "I am grateful that I am peaceful and happy", and "I am grateful that I pray everyday". The truth is, silly as it may sound, words have power and what you speak, you will become! If you have been used to you calling yourself names, putting yourself down and demonstrating lack of belief in yourself, this may be hard for you. But if you have to fake it for now, that's okay. Once you start speaking this new truth about yourself, your mind will believe it to be so; then you'll **naturally** begin taking action to acquire your vision, and you will receive the results you desire in your body. Here is the simple equation:

$$\begin{array}{c} \text{Be Grateful} \\ + \text{Believe} + \\ \text{Take Action} \\ = \text{Receive} \end{array}$$

You have learned to use your words to build up instead of tear down laying a new foundation of belief in yourself as worthy and successful, and you have set a vision for the woman you are destined to become. Reflect on her everyday, keep her always in your mind, and in time you'll find that you are making the types of choices that this free, healthy, happy Vixen would make! Coming up on the road ahead, you will encounter situations and circumstances that trigger you to make poor choices, but you'll also learn how to develop the tools to overcome them. You'll learn how to drop the excuses for good, and get back on the road if you've stalled out.

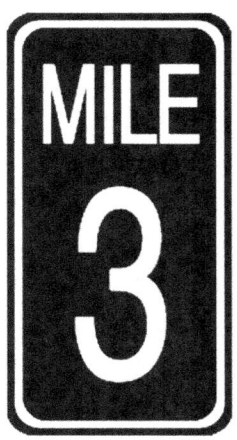

ACTION STEPS

- Create your Vixen Vision Board (Your travel brochure)
- Set a destination on your GPS by writing out your goals for Mind, Body and Spirit in your journal
- Add to your current mirroring exercises by practicing saying out loud what you like about your "future self" as if it were real today.
- Continue with part 1 and now add part 2 of the Gratitude Wheel to your daily routine, by writing words of thanks in your journal each night for the woman you will become.
- Continue following the *High Octane Diet*
- Continue with your exercise regime
- Weigh in daily or weekly and track your changes.
- Drink 8-10 cups of water each day

Week 4

Looking Under The Hood...

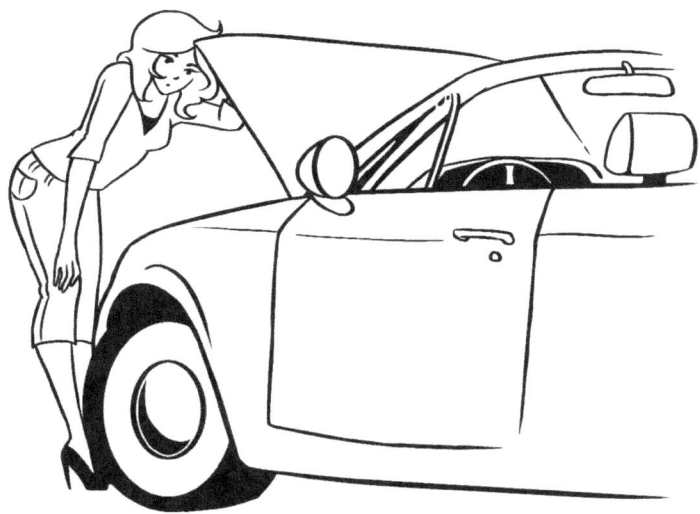

Sometimes we find ourselves getting "stuck" with our weight-loss. We believe that we're eating healthy, exercising, and doing all of the right things but the scales and our pants size don't seem to move. Why is that? I've done it myself... gone months "eating right and exercising" with no results! That is the reason why it is so important to track what you eat, when you eat, how you eat, your emotions, what you're doing for exercise...everything. It may seem like just another thing "to do", but I assure you it is for good reason. When we track what we've been doing, it gives us a log to refer to when something isn't going right; where we may have gotten off course. And many times we'll find that the problem is that we're not doing what we think we're doing! We are making up excuses more often than not, and we are ignoring the warning lights when they occur. It's like driving down the road and a warning light comes on that says you need to put oil in your car, and you ignore it because (here comes your excuse) you're in a hurry to get somewhere, and you promise to look at it later. "Later" comes and goes, and you continue to ignore the warning light. Then one day, your engine stops completely. Had you only taken a few minutes to pull over on the side of the road, look under the hood, and add some oil… you would still have a fine running engine. This week we're going to look under your hood… in your head…to see what triggers you to get off course, and the excuses you make to avoid taking care of your health.

Warning lights

Did you know that over 75% of people eat for emotional reasons? Here's some of the "reasons" that people, women in particularly, eat (besides being hungry):

- Because they are socializing and want to "fit in" and do what everyone else is doing.
- Because they are bored, angry, stressed, anxious, depressed, and worried.
- Because they feel inadequate, especially around certain other women.

- Because they turn to food for comfort, to fill the need to be loved.

If you are one of those 75% of people that eat for emotional reasons, I know how you are feeling, because I have struggled with it myself. A few years ago, I took a break one afternoon from work and met my husband at our favorite Thai restaurant for lunch. The food was great, but during lunch we had a heavy conversation about money. I walked out of the restaurant feeling physically full… a little overstuffed, actually. On the way back to work, only a few blocks from the restaurant, I spotted an Italian Ice stand. It was really weird; because I felt a hunger pang at the same time I noticed the stand, so I made the split second decision to pull into the parking lot. Luckily, before jumping out of the car I stopped myself. "Why am I doing this?" I wondered. So, I thought about what was going through my head only moments before turning into the lot. Then, it happened. I experienced my first "Ah-ha" moment when it came to discovering one of my triggers! It was the "money conversation". So then, I took it a step further…I asked myself how those thoughts made me feel – anxious. Asking myself what I had been doing, how I had been feeling, and what I was thinking enabled me to pause and stop myself from diving head-first into a tall, cold, orange-cream flavored Italian ice. I had just finished a meal, so it was illogical for me to be physically hungry. I realized that my brain must have been seeking comfort and distraction from the uneasy "money conversation" still going on in my head. Giving myself that moment to stop and think is just what I needed to make a rational decision. To get my mind (and stomach) off of the Italian ice, I knew that I had to re-direct my senses and thoughts onto something else with such strong intent, that all other thoughts would go away. So, I used one of my favorite gear-shifters. "Gear-shifters" are a distraction tool that I use to help move my focus and intention on to something else. In order to avoid the sweet temptation, I stared up at the blue sky, and focused in on how the blue in the sky contrasted with the green treetops. I zoomed in on that color contrast so intently that my financial anxiety just melted away. Once I felt calm and in control, I found my "hunger" was gone, the stomach pangs went away, and I went back to work, minus the unnecessary calories and sugar. So here is the sequence of what could have happened:

Trigger —money conversation. Thoughts —not enough money. Emotions – anxiety, worry. Action – eat sweets. Emotions – guilt. Action – eat more. Results – gain weight.

And here is the sequence of what actually happened:

Trigger – money conversation. Thoughts – not enough money. Emotions – anxiety, worry. Action – stop, reflect, breathe, use gear shifter to get in "the moment" and calm down. Emotion – peace. Action – move forward with my day. Results – avoid excess sugar, reduce stress, and enjoy the day. Long term results – lose weight.

So, as you can see, you can make a choice. But first, you need to know your triggers. Then you need to have a plan of attack when they arise. What are your triggers? Think about it…These triggers are your warning lights, letting you know that something is very wrong. Identifying exactly what sets you off will allow you to become more aware of those times when they occur.

My Italian Ice story illustrates an interesting point – though I had just eaten, and acknowledged to myself that I was full, when presented with the Italian Ice, I experienced real hunger pangs. That was a physical sign that I was hungry. However, I wasn't really hungry at all! In fact, my subconscious mind guided my stomach to tell me that the sweets would take away the feelings of anxiety. If I could get my mind onto food, I could get it off of money. Had I only paid attention to the hunger pangs, and not stopped to think about it, I may have eaten the Italian ice. Sometimes hunger pangs are real, and sometimes they are a warning light; an indicator that something deeper is going on. So it's important to learn how to *really* listen to our body. My subconscious mind misled my stomach, indeed as an attempt to distract me from my anxiety. But my body never lied to me, and neither will yours lie to you. Just like a fever blister is a signal or warning light of an underlying illness, stressor, or infection, my hunger pang was a physical warning light of my underlying emotional worry over money. And my body was telling me that. Yours, too will tell you exactly what it needs, when it needs it, and when it's enough or too much. After all, what do you think your lingering fat is? It's also a signal... it's your body telling you that something else is chronically going on inside and its time for you to investigate. If you are showing symptoms of anything, whether that be obesity, sleeplessness, anger, chronic illness, etc... yes, it's good to go to a functional medicine practitioner to run tests, but you also need to learn how to trust yourself and how to listen to your body effectively to see what's really going on. You need to look under the hood! My hunger pain was merely a sign that something deeper was going on. And when I took the time to think about it, I figured it out. So, how do you read YOUR body signals to avoid making an excuse and getting off track? Its actually very simple: You SLOW down your reactions, your thoughts, and your impulses...focus on getting in the moment, breathe, and relax. Then take the time to analyze everything by using your power of reasoning.

In addition to the triggers that spark your emotional eating response, there are also a variety of physical triggers that can cause you to eat junk food, or overeat altogether when you are not truly hungry. Hormonal changes can trigger you to overeat, specifically sweets. I mean... how many of us can't claim to have had a powerful desire for a Hershey bar at "that time" of the month? And if you're like me, going through even early stages of menopause was like having PMS the entire month long (until I had tests done and began using bio-identical hormone replacement therapy) Couple that with a sedentary stressful job, and it's no wonder I got fat!! Another trigger may be your chemical addiction to processed carbohydrates. Perhaps it was difficult for you to cut way down on sugar and excess carbs a few weeks ago, and in that case you know exactly what I am talking about. Those first couple of days may have been extremely challenging, but now it doesn't seem like a very big deal. That's because you were experiencing symptoms of withdrawal, not unlike a drug user would! Another cause of overeating is lack of adequate sleep. If you are tired, your body may crave the quick energy found in sweets and carbohydrates, which will make you feel temporarily more awake, though what you really need is more rest. In that same vain, the signal that tells us we are thirsty is similar to hunger cues, and often we eat when what we really need is a tall glass of water. Are you eating when you should be sleeping or drinking more? No wonder you don't feel well! Finally, a simple trigger is just the sight of unhealthy food, whether it is stocked in your pantry or you spy your favorite fast food place on the way home from work; either of these can trigger you to salivate like Pavlov's dog. These are all physical triggers that cause a false sense of hunger. It is equivalent to the fuel light going on, when all the while you have a full tank of gas – you don't physically need it, but you've been conditioned to believe that you do. Let's talk a little more about where that "conditioning" came from and how we can change it.

Many times this emotional connection to eating food stems from your early childhood conditioning. Remember going to a birthday party when you were young? What was served? Pizza, soda, candy, and cake! However, many of these paradigms have continued into adult-hood. As adults, our social events revolve around food and alcohol, which most of the time includes sweets and processed carbohydrates. So our subconscious mind automatically associates pleasure (parties) with food and alcohol (which is high in sugar content too).

If we are stressed, angry, or worried, we reach for the one thing that our subconscious mind associates with pleasure, in order to "cure" the unpleasant emotions...food. In order to shift this paradigm, we need to be able to recognize these subconscious triggers. Once we do, that's half the battle. Just like I know now that heated discussions about money is one of my triggers. So, if one of these conversations randomly comes up, I'm prepared to shift my gears. We all have patterns of behavior in life. Some are good, and some could use a shift. No worries, though... throughout this whole 12-week process you are learning various tools to help shift those paradigms and create a healthier, more passionate life.

Unfortunately we cannot remove all the stress or challenging circumstances from your life, but we can develop new ways of dealing with them rather than using food. The purpose of food is to keep you alive and healthy, it is not therapy. Identifying your triggers and breaking them down to the root cause is absolutely critical to becoming a healthy and happy *Vixen Unleashed*. So I want you to go to your journal, and take a few moments to record every physical and emotional trigger that you can come up with. You may not hit them all right now, so always carry a little notepad, your journal or your smart phone with you at all times, to record each new trigger you identify, as they arise. Just knowing and acknowledging them ahead of time will ring a little mental bell every time you encounter the situation again.

Here are some examples of triggers and potential reactions to them: When you fight with your spouse, do you run to the cupboard? When the boss demands that you work overtime and you are already maxed out, do you hit the stash of M&Ms in the bottom drawer? Does a conversation with your mother cause you to eat the leftover birthday cake? Each of these triggers points to a person... but realistically; *people* are not your triggers. It's more likely something that they commonly say or do, or situations that you associate with them, which stir up your emotions. To dig into the specifics of what those triggers are, and more importantly, determine the cause of those triggers, you have to be prepared to ask yourself some questions, and answer honestly. The next time you find yourself elbow deep in a bag of chips, I want you to pause and ask yourself four questions that will uncover EXACTLY what has made you overeat unhealthy food:

1. What is/was happening in my life today?
2. What exactly was I thinking right before I binged/overate/made unhealthy food choices?
3. What emotions have I been feeling today?
4. What deep, underlying fears could be causing me to experience these emotions and feelings?

Here's an example scenario: Let's say you work in sales and your boss comes into your office one afternoon and demands that you get your numbers up. You arrive home from work in the evening thinking about how much you despise your boss, reliving the conversation over and over in your head, and as you walk into the house you that your son has left a package of Girl Scout cookies on the counter. Without thinking, you sit down and an entire sleeve of Girl Scout cookies. Afterward you may feel angry with yourself and beat yourself up (emotionally) for your lack of self-control. But instead of wasting time with this self-abuse, what if you took a minute to ask the four questions? Once you are aware of what might be going on, you'd grab your journal or notepad and jot down what you discovered:

- Triggers - Your boss approached you with pressures to perform better (emotional trigger) and there was a box of cookies on the table (physical trigger).

- Thoughts – I despise my boss; he has no idea how hard I work; I can't do anymore than I already do; I'm not appreciated at work; doesn't he see the value in me?
- Emotions - Anxiety, frustration, worry, anger.
- Fears – I'm afraid if I don't perform better at work, I'll lose my job, have no income and not be able to support my family or possibly become homeless.

It is ideal that you stop yourself before you eat the foods you'd prefer not to, and ask these questions. But if you didn't catch yourself in time – do not be too hard on yourself. See it as an opportunity for growth, and another chance to understand the root cause of what has always made you reach to food, instead of a healthier alternative to nurse your feelings or comfort you in times of distress. What *is* a safer and healthier way to wade through difficult feelings instead of eating them away? Let's pop the trunk and take out your tool box, and I'll show you what you need to get back on the road.

GET OUT THE TOOLBOX

If you have the right tools, you can overcome virtually any car trouble on your journey to Freedom. You are going to learn how to counteract each and every one of those triggers on your list, in not just one way, but multiple ways so you are always ready no matter where you are at that moment. Realistically, you cannot remove your triggers, but you can change your reaction to them. For example, there will always be conversations about money with my spouse. It's inevitable. However, I can learn how to change my reactions to any feelings of discomfort that arise from those conversations. There will always be difficult people and situations in life that can be challenging to deal with, but with the right tools, we can change how we respond to those uncomfortable feelings.

Twenty-five years ago I was a smoker who wanted to quit. To stop smoking I chose to use a gear-shifter. I decided that every time I wanted a cigarette, I first had to run for 5 minutes! So nearly ten times a day I would jump on the treadmill or run around the block. When I would start running, my lungs would open up and I would breathe in large gulps of clean, fresh air. (Or sometimes I would have coughing fits!) Endorphins would release into my blood stream from the exertion and I'd start to feel energetic and happy. All of these physical sensations reminded me of why I was quitting in the first place, so I couldn't have chosen a better gear-shifter! Eventually I was able to quit completely and instead of gaining weight like many do when they give up smoking, I actually lost it! This tool of using exercise as my distraction method works great for weight loss. What gear-shifters can you think of to help ward off self-sabotaging behaviors when your triggers arise?

Let's revisit your triggers list. For every trigger you have uncovered, you are going to come up with some options to help you shift into a new direction. There are many different techniques that you can employ, so you will have to decide what works best for you. Each time you are triggered to eat and you have determined that the hunger isn't real, feel free to employ one of the strategies below, but I encourage you to come up with your own as well! How about inventing a silly ritual like clapping your hands three times, or stamping your foot to put the brakes on and snap yourself out of it? It is almost like a stiff slap across the face, waking you up and giving you time to think rationally. Your distraction technique might be turning on some music, writing in your journal, or whipping off 20 jumping jacks. You can divert your attention to positive thoughts by repeating a mantra such as "Food is not love" or "I am worth more than this", or "eating this does not serve me". You can pull out your Vixen Vision board and remind yourself of why you are taking this journey, and how important your goals are to you. You can post reminders on little sticky notes that say something like: "Is this helping me reach my goal?" on your refrigerator or other key danger zones around your home, work or car, where you will be able to read and repeat them in times of temptation. However, even if you use one of the above mentioned gear-shifters to get you away from the pantry and stop you from diving into the cookies, once you've stepped away from the situation, and "snapped out of it", so to speak...I want you to practice slowing down your thoughts, movements, breathing, and actions and allow all of your senses to zone in on the now, and live in the moment. This technique is not only to help you avoid eating cookies; the more that you practice this, the better everything in your life will be. Think of it as relaxing yourself into the face of your emotions, by doing a gentle 3 part breathing exercise - breathe your nostrils, slowly filling first your abdomen with your breath, then your ribs, and finally your chest, then hold it for 10 seconds. Follow that with a slow exhale, pressing the air through your lips. Then, once you have calmed down, zero in on each of your senses; smell, sounds, sights, touch, and tastes. Just notice.... *being*.

All of these tools are designed to give you the space to calm down and focus on something other than the immediate gratification of food. You may want to have several different gear-shifters ready to employ, depending on your circumstances. After all, a stressful business meeting with a tempting platter of donuts on the table is no place to do 30 squats! But repeating a mantra silently may be just the ticket in that situation.

You've learned to identify triggers, thoughts, emotions and fears. You've learned how you can use gear-shifters to change your emotional direction and get your mind off of using food as medication to soothe your pain. More importantly, you've learned how to slow down, breathe, focus on your senses and live in the moment to dissipate the pain and avoid self-sabotage. However, when those triggers arise, even when you know what they are, and you have your gear-shifters ready to go... there is still the chance that you may stall!

STALLING

If your car is constantly stalling out, eventually it will just quit and you'll never make it to your destination. Likewise, if you are constantly stalling with excuses in your weight loss program, eventually you will just quit and never reach your health and weight loss goals.

Everyone has excuses – reasons or stories as to why they can't do or follow through with something. So, what are yours? Do you make excuses for not exercising? Is it that you are too tired, too busy, you have a headache or your body hurts, you don't have enough time, or maybe you just don't like to exercise? Or, perhaps you have stories as to why you aren't eating healthfully. Here are some great ones: "Eating healthy is too expensive", "My family loves junk food so it's always in my house", "I don't have time to prepare meals in advance", or "I hate vegetables". In order to stop "stalling", you're going to have to be honest with yourself and admit when you're making excuses. It's easy to convince yourself that your excuses are valid. But, nine times out of ten, they are not.

Here is a tactic you can use to determine whether or not you're making excuses, or if your reason for not following through is actually valid: Think of all the reasons why you don't follow through with a healthful lifestyle plan, and list them in your journal. Every time that you catch yourself getting ready to make an excuse, pull out your journal, grab a pen and add that excuse to the list. Next to each of your excuses, come up with an action or thought to change direction. For example if your excuse is "I have no time to exercise" then solutions may include re-purposing your lunch hour, getting up 20 minutes earlier, or skipping your late night TV show. If your excuse is that you don't have time to cook healthy food then a solution may be precooking lunches and snacks for the week and freezing them, or learning to eat and enjoy more raw foods. Logically thinking through an excuse may prove to you that it is not actually a legitimate reason, or perhaps it may enable you to view the problem in a new way. Let's say you are too tired to exercise because you didn't get enough sleep last night. But you know that if you exercise it causes you to sleep much better, so if you can push through the fatigue today, you'll sleep great tonight and have more energy to work out harder tomorrow. If you really want something, you will make time. Maybe you need to re-evaluate your priorities, and put your health and well being at the top of the list, where it belongs. If you can find ways to counteract all of the excuses you have, you'll run out of reasons to hold back any longer, and soon you'll be flying along the interstate, as the woman you were born to be!

Now that you know what to do when you have engine trouble, you are equipped for the rest of the journey; you'll be able to overcome excuses, read the warning lights when trouble is on the horizon and get back on the straight and narrow quickly. Next week you will learn how to navigate a fork in the road — when a critical decision can make all the difference!

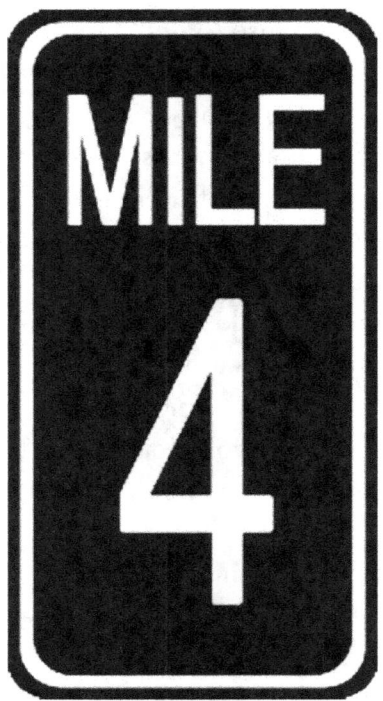

ACTION STEPS

- Make a list of your triggers and "gear-shifters" to counteract them
- List all of your excuses, and action steps to overcome them
- Continue to practice parts 1 & 2 of the Gratitude Wheel and mirroring exercises
- Continue with the *High Octane Diet*
- Continue with your exercise regime
- Weigh in daily or weekly and track your changes.
- Drink 8-10 cups of water each day

Week 5

Choosing Which Way To Go.

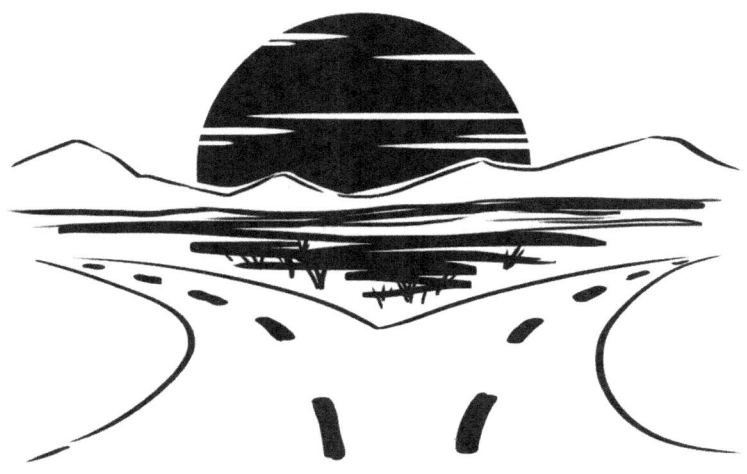

Congratulations, you've reached week five and are well on your way! The first month of any new practice is always the toughest, but you have started making new choices that soon will develop into good habits! Every choice you make, both in weight-loss and in life, determines the direction you go in and ultimately, where you end up. Interestingly, the more personal growth and positive change you seek, the more decisions you will have to make. However, those decisions will be easier made if you know two things:

1. How to strategize and plan in advance for any mishaps.
2. How to read and follow your own inner compass.

Anytime you make a decision to make changes in your life, whether that's a career change, or losing 15 pounds, it's always best to begin with a strategy and refer to it often, to help keep you on the success track. There may come a time when you reach a fork in the road, and you'll have to make a split-second decision. Its times like these when your plan will be the key to you pressing on, in the right direction. Sometimes there are bumps in the road that require you to deviate from the established course and take an alternate route; you might even find that it's not always the more obvious one that will get you where you really want to go. This is when you must rely on your inner compass to determine the best direction for you. Last week we discussed the importance of recognizing your triggers, and using gear-shifters to help you avoid a possible collision with binging or eating junk food. This week you'll be given tools to help you make better choices throughout your journey on Interstate Vixen12. You'll be learning different routes to help get you to the same destination, Freedom.

BUILD IT INTO YOUR LIFESTYLE

When I began my personal road-trip, changing my diet was much easier than changing my exercise habits. It wasn't that I hated exercise. I knew that it felt good once I did it. As a busy professional, who was dedicated to her work both at the office and inside the home…to me, exercise was just too time consuming. In my mind, there was not enough time in the day for anything else; especially for exercise! I don't know on how many different occasions, I would begin a

60-minute exercise DVD, only to stop 15 minutes into it. I would get overwhelmed just thinking about it taking up too much precious time! How ironic! Cognitively, I knew that exercising would give me the energy and clarity to actually increase my productivity and make my day go smoother! But the fear and anxiety from the idea of it interfering with my "to-do" list would always get the best of me. So, in order to end that crazy notion, I first decided that I would trick my mind into stop thinking of exercise as a means to lose weight. I would think of it as a means to help eliminate stress, allowing me to work with more clarity and efficiency. It wasn't like I was really lying to myself. That was the truth! Exercise would increase my endorphins, thus boost my energy and help me be more productive! I was just taking a different approach to my *perception* of working out, to one that my "workaholic-self" would be more receptive to. By doing that, exercise actually became a *part of* my to-do list, which would make my workday flow better, rather than being something *on top of* my to-do list. (See how changing the phraseology in my head made exercise a good thing?)

Additionally, I decided to commit to only *one* 45-minute exercise DVD per week for that first week, in which I also enlisted a friend to do with me. I also promised myself to simply begin "moving" more, doing something I enjoyed. I knew the importance of balance in life, so I figured why not make my "play time" incorporate movement! So, for 20 minutes a few times each week I would do something fun — dancing in my living room, jogging with the dog, or playing a dance video game with my son. I enjoyed these activities, so they never felt like exercise. While doing some of the lighter forms of movement, like cleaning house or taking a gentle walk outside in the evening, I listened to an affirmation CD that I had created. This empowered me and helped re-condition my mind-set so I began to look forward to exercising and nourishing my body. Within a few weeks, I added a second focused 45-minute exercise session, in which I did with a different friend. Having someone to be accountable to, gave me more incentive to get my workout in each week, plus it gave me an excuse to hang out with my girlfriends, also a very much-needed thing to incorporate into good self-care. I continued to add exercise like this gradually overtime until a time came when I was getting regular exercise 5 days per week. I never felt overwhelmed or resentful, because I made these changes incrementally, and I made exercise a part of my life, rather than just something else I *had* to do. When faced with making a choice of exercise or no exercise, I found a way to incorporate it as part of my work life and my social life, and I made the changes slowly to ensure that could stick to them and build good habits.

TURN BY TURN

When you drive somewhere, it is rarely in a straight line, and you most likely will have to make turns. Each turn brings you closer to your destination. If you were magic, you could just blink your eyes and be there! However, without going through the process of discovering your authentic self and working through the underlying cause of your weight-gain, the magic would soon wear off and you would end up back home, in the Comfort Zone. Does this sound familiar? I mean, have you ever busted tail for a few months to lose the weight, only to see it return? That's why it's important to implement change one step at a time. This way, you can build habits. There may come a time, once you've established great habits that you'd like to up your game and do a 90-day challenge and take your health to the next level! But until you firmly establish good self care, self-love and healthier habits, even a 90-day challenge that you "win" might very well set you up with another "I lost it, then gained it back" scenario. So, it's important to go through this process to help you gain inner strength to create that outer beauty, before you dive into something you're not truly ready for. The only way you will get to true Freedom is through unleashing your inner Vixen and following the map turn by turn. Sometimes it might seem that you're just taking baby steps and you want to hurry and get to the finish line! But remember the hare and the tortoise? This is a great example of how taking your time and doing it right will make you a winner in the long run, and end years of frustration for you in the future! You might still be far away from your ultimate goal-weight. But this is exactly how you will get to your destination - with a string of small, and seemingly insignificant (but realistically, very powerful) choices, and actions. It may feel like your tiny little action steps at the end of each mile-marker are never going to get you to your bigger picture, and you might even consider brushing them aside to focus on something else, like working out harder and eating less! But aren't those tactics you've used before? Where did they get you? We live in a society of instant gratification. So when you don't have that immediate satisfaction on the scale or in your jeans, you'll tend to either give up right then and there, or go like gangbusters, and then give up a few weeks down the road. We all want immediate results. However, with the *Vixen Unleashed* program, by implementing your action steps and practicing them daily, your results will go much deeper and be much more gratifying than a just the number on the scale. So, take heart and trust. Keep at it, and little steps, made consistently over time, will create a radical change, both inside and out. This is called compounding gain, and it is one of the founding principals of the *Vixen Unleashed* program.

Let me give you an example of compounding gain at work. Let's say we have sisters, both married with children, and both overweight. Sister A decides there is nothing she can adjust about her lifestyle, thinking she is too busy to change, and resigns herself to being over-weight. Sister B is just as busy as sister A, and daunted by the challenge of losing weight. However, she is unwilling to sit idol and allow her-self to live in an unhealthy body. So she decides that 5 nights per week during her favorite prime-time sitcom, she will walk at 3 MPH on the treadmill for 30 minutes (notice how she made it *part of* her routine). She also wants to break her sugar and caffeine addiction to soda, and decides to exchange the 20 oz. bottle of cola she drinks every after-noon for sparkling water. Since the changes aren't significant, she is able to stick with it. Of course, after a month not much has happened. Sister B is still overweight, though she feels a bit more energetic, and is sleeping better now that she is getting a modest amount of exercise and kicked her caffeine habit. The scale only moved a tiny bit, but the lifestyle changes feel right, so she sticks with it. Both sisters kept up with this program, and revisiting them in a year is a huge eye opener. Sister A is still overweight, unhappy and feels powerless. But sister B, who burned 150 extra calories per day through walking, and 240 calories per day by removing the soda, is now 36 lbs lighter! All she did was make 2 small manageable changes, and she stuck with them. It really is that simple! Remember this equation:

> Smart daily choices + time + con-sistency = big gains.

But this example is a bit unrealistic. What is more likely to happen is that once sister B started seeing positive changes, such as sleeping better, having more energy and losing a little weight, she would have stepped up her workouts. Perhaps she made one more change - to exchange her bowl of breakfast cereal for egg whites, and she wound up losing even more weight. She felt better about herself, and her intimate relationship with her husband improved, increasing their marital happiness. Without the sugar crash in the afternoon, she was more productive at work, her boss took notice and she got a raise. The family used the extra money to go on vacation and spend time together. She was able to make a fresh connection with her kids as they took an active vacation - riding bikes, snorkeling and going on sightseeing hikes. This is called a ripple effect. Rarely do you make a change that has no impact on other areas of your life. If you make a positive change the ripple effect will be positive, if it's a negative change then that negativity will infiltrate many areas of life. By making a few small smart choices and sticking to them, Sister B changed the course of her life. There is a strong chance that Sister A didn't stay the same either – she continued to overeat, and do nothing and her health and happiness just deteriorated further.

This principle is a thread through the entire *Vixen Unleashed* program – completing your weekly action steps, while still following through daily on the steps from previous weeks. Doing so methodically and consistently will take you exactly where you want to go, to a life of health and freedom.

HAVING A BACK-UP PLAN

Often what derails our healthy eating and exercising habits is just one small choice. Perhaps you were on a diet before, and got invited out to dinner. You had a great month on the program and were feeling good about yourself. The dinner date was later than you'd normally eat, so by the time you were seated you were famished. You had every intention of eating light and healthy tonight, but when the waiter brings the bread you tell yourself, "okay, just one piece". Pretty soon it is half the basket, and hey – since you messed up already, might as well go for the whole enchilada and get the heavy meal and the dessert. It's just one night! But the next morning you wake up ashamed, and bloated and disappointed in yourself, and to console yourself, you have 2 of the blueberry muffins you made for your kids, instead of the usual egg white and veggie omelet. Two weeks later you are firmly back into your old habits, and wondering how that simple fork in the road caused you to change direction and head back to the comfort zone. What happened? It was actually a series of bumps in the road. Let's take a look:

1. Your dinner date was late, and you became famished.
2. You were in a situation that stimulated your senses, which enticed you want bread, and when compounded with your massive hunger, you dove into a piece of bread.
3. The processed carbohydrate and gluten created a physical desire for more of the same. So you ate more bread.
4. You felt ashamed that you caved in and felt disappointed in yourself for your lack of "willpower" and to wash away that shame, you ate more bread.

5. You told yourself "It's just one night", to help cover up your <u>feelings</u> of failure.
6. The next day you punished yourself for being a "failure" and sought comfort and love from more of the same.

This type of behavior instills into your mind that you are unworthy, not good enough, and a failure. Which was worse? Eating the piece of bread or your harmful negative self-talk? I'm here to say it was the latter of the two. But before we go there… let's take a look at some ways that you could have prevented all of this from happening.

1. Eating something every 2-3 hours will help stop that feeling of being "famished". When planning to go out for dinner, eat something healthy and filling before you go… even if it's only 1 ½ hours after your last small meal. In other words, let's say you ate at 3pm, and expected your date at 4:30pm, which would have put you at eating at the restaurant somewhere between 5-6. Had he shown up and everything went as planned, that would have been perfect! But when 4:30 rolled around and he wasn't there… that's the time you pull out a pre-made plate of veggies and some hummus to dip them into, or you make a protein shake and drink it. The next thing you'd want to do is to pack a handful of nuts in your purse. Eating just 6 or 7 nuts 30 minutes before your meal with a glass of water, will cut down that hunger pang that can cause you to overeat, or make poorer choices. Taking a handful of nuts will be good though, because what if after dinner, your date decided to do an impromptu movie? You would then already be prepared to eat a few nuts during the movie rather than a buttery bucket of popcorn!
2. Let's say you ate beforehand so you weren't famished… but the smell of the freshly baked bread was getting to you! When

the waiter comes out, kindly let him know that you prefer no bread this evening. Or.. if your date wants the bread and your smelling senses are beginning to get the best of you, then SLOW DOWN and take a few deep breaths, relaxing into the moment. Think about the wonderful company you have and that you want to enjoy "breaking bread" with him, then breathe… and allow yourself a piece of bread, knowing that it is not going to hurt you one bit… and when you eat that one piece of bread, savor every single morsel… tasting it, smelling it, feeling the texture in your mouth. When you are calm and relaxed, using all of your senses to enjoy the moment, you enjoy the moment! And you also increase the digestive juices in your body to help assimilate the food better and improve your digestion for that meal by up to 40%! That, within itself will negate the additional calories you just had! Now, if you have determined that you ARE gluten intolerant or sensitive, and then just continue to breathe deeply, eat a few more nuts, and get truly in the moment of the conversation with this awesome guy! Remember… Live Sensually!

3. Now, let's say that you decided to pick up an additional piece of bread. The BEST things you can do at that point is relax, breathe, smile and ENJOY the food SLOWLY and live sensually in the moment with your date!

4. Simply visualize yourself pushing out any negative thinking with each exhale of breath, and as you inhale take a moment to imagine a white light of positive energy filling your body. In with the positive, out with the negative. I'd rather you eat a piece of bread with peace and serenity, with all of your senses involved in the pleasure of the conversation and the tastes of the food, then have you beat yourself up for having a bite.

5. The other thing you want to steer clear of, is making the decision to NOT eat the bread, and then spend the rest of the

evening focusing on how much you want it but can't have it, rather than sitting there enjoying the time with your date! That would be far worse for you than eating the bread. The stress that you would put on yourself from this mental battle *alone* will hold on to your weight tighter than it would, had you eaten the bread in the first place. Just know that this is all part of YOUR process of healing and accept that this is just you, and you are amazing! Surrender your thoughts as you breathe in deeply and ask your Divine Feminine within to take those fears away!

Here are a few other tips to help you be more prepared and make better choices when planning to dine out...

- Check out the menu online ahead of time if possible, so you know what healthy meal options you have.
- Order your meats/poultry/fish with light seasoning and grilled or baked.
- Try to avoid casseroles.
- Ask for salad with no croutons, and dressing on the side, preferably olive oil or vinaigrette type dressings. Only add a few Tablespoons to the salad.
- Ask for a double order of steamed or roasted non-starchy veggies, rather than one order of veggies and a big baked potato! There is no harm in eating a little extra broccoli one night!
- If the portions are large, ask the waiter right away for a take-home box so you can divide your meal in half and save the rest for lunch the next day!
- And most importantly, eat slowly and eat SENSUALLY, using all of your senses to enjoy your food, your company, and your experience!

One bump in the road does not have to be the end of the road for your weight loss journey. Be prepared for anything that comes up, to arm you with a plan that makes it easier to reach your desired goals. If you have a plan in advance, those split second decisions will be good ones, and will prevent you from going down a road that takes you further away from your destination.

TIME IS ON YOUR SIDE — WITH A STRATEGY IN PLACE!

So, now you understand the value in advance planning, and how it will help you make better choices, and possibly prevent you from slipping back into old habits and returning to the Comfort Zone. But you're probably thinking to yourself, "Who's got the time to plan and prepare like that?" Being a busy woman, I understand how you can feel overwhelmed at times; as if there is no time left in your day for anything. Part of going through this program is learning how to let go of that overwhelmed feeling, and that there is not enough time. Those are both fear driven thoughts that don't serve you. When you find those thoughts entering in to your mind, practice sensual living. By utilizing all of your senses to be *aware* and live in the moment, you will help get those untrue thoughts to dissipate! There IS enough time, but sometimes we need a little help in managing it so it flows more smoothly in our lives. In the next several weeks we will be tackling these issues a little more deeply. For now, I ask you to trust that your Higher Power has your back… and when you begin feeling overwhelmed, and out of time… Breathe, relax, and slow down your thinking and actions. SLOW DOWN and practice sensual living!

When you believe that there is a lack of time, then there will be. So practice believing the opposite - that there is PLENTY of time! Remember our self-talk we used? That doesn't only apply to your looks. It applies to every day living! Using affirmations is one of the best ways of making things right in your life. And instead of saying the reasons that you "can't" do something, then start saying the things that you "can" do. Remember what we did last week with your excuses? Okay... so let's say that one of your excuses is "there is not enough time in my day to prepare food in advance". What is the opposite of that? How "can" I make this work for me, and what can I do to make the time for food preparation?

Start by coming up with a strategy. Choose one or two times a week to do major prep work and grocery shopping. This will help ensure that you always have plenty of healthy snacks on hand. I will usually put together a few containers pre-filled with nuts, hummus or hardboiled eggs, so when I have to run an errand, I have something I can throw into my purse and go! Being ready with a snack is ideal, but what happens if you forgot – and you are at the shopping mall or out on the town? Nearly every place you go – even the fast food places, has salads these days. If you are desperate, you can always get a grilled chicken sandwich and toss out the bun. There is virtually always some healthy option available, though you may have to be creative. After you make the healthier choice, and your hunger is gone, you will feel so proud and empowered; it will drive you to do it the next time too.

Other strategies will include handling a social function, a party, the holidays, or a birthday. Those events can be a little intimidating when you're on a diet. Once again, eating something before you go, and taking along a little snack, will save you from propping yourself by the food table all night. More importantly, it helps to think of the evening as a social occasion, and focus on spending time in good conversation with people you care about, instead of trying to eat as much cake as you can. Oftentimes at a party that serves alcohol, people will encourage you to drink because they want you to relax and have fun. If you do dare to indulge, keep in mind that white wine and mixed drinks are filled with sugar, so I recommend enjoying one glass of red wine. Or, better yet, have a club soda with a splash of cranberry juice for color, and a lime. No one needs to know what you are drinking, and as soon as they see that drink in your hand, they'll stop asking you to have a drink! And if you are still not very comfortable in your own skin...Instead of worrying that you will be a target of attention for your appearance, take time with dressing yourself so you feel good. Play up your assets with flattering clothes and accessories that make you feel your best. You will be more outgoing and be having so much fun, you'll forget all about the cheese tray. Laugh, have a good time and enjoy the party - Sensually!

And don't forget to have a strategy if you travel for work or go on vacations. Traveling, whether for work or pleasure is a very common excuse to slack off on healthy living. Long hours, airports, plane rides and the desire for relaxation are all reasons you might give to ditch your program. Who hasn't come back from vacation with 5 lbs to lose from too much indulgent food, drinks, and lounging? But travel doesn't have to be an excuse to take a vacation from the new life you are living! If you are prepared, you can keep the engine running strong and make even more progress away from home. Nearly every hotel has a fitness facility these days, but to be sure – take the time to look into it when you book your stay. If there isn't a facility – look into gyms that may be in your destination city. Many fitness centers such as Bally's, LA Fitness, or Planet Fitness have centers all over the US, and your local membership may be good nationwide. (Of course if you're going to Orlando, Florida, you can also visit Vixen Fitness!) With the Internet, you have every opportunity to scout out great places to eat and play on any trip. Vacations are a time for rejuvenation — and what could be more rejuvenating than yoga on the beach, a little snorkeling or a bike ride on the boardwalk? Balance your downtime on your trip, with "up" time as well — where you are exploring the sites and using your body. Your V12 Turbo Boost exercises can be done anywhere, and is a great option in a hotel. You can pack resistance bands or your favorite workout DVD, as well as do basic calisthenics right in your hotel room to start or end each day off right. Be proactive! I had every excuse in the world not to exercise or eat right as a flight attendant, but I made it work. And remember to be gentle with yourself. If you do find yourself indulging a little on vacation with some chocolate or wine, enjoy it, taste it, and be a part of it, and then just throw in a few extra minutes on your morning beach walk the next day!

You've learned about many different scenarios where you will have to make a split second decision. And you've also learned several different routes to help keep you on the road to Freedom. Having strategies and back-up plans will be one key to your success in weight loss. But if you reach a moment when you just can't seem to figure out which way to go on your journey, don't forget to use your inner compass. You can always rely on that to help steer you in the right direction. You are well on your way to being the Vixen you've been dreaming of, and deserve a pat on the back for all of your hard work! Make sure to keep reminding yourself in the mirror and your journal that you have a lot to be grateful for - things you have now, and dreams you haven't yet realized. Up ahead you will discover how to stop, look, and listen to what your mind and body and spirit are telling you.

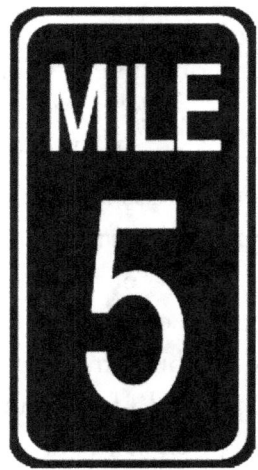

Action Steps

- Head out to a favorite restaurant this week to practice your knowledge of which way to go. Plan ahead using your new strategies
- Be gentle on yourself!
- Write in your journal some of the ways that you are going to handle forks in the road
- Continue with your Gratitude Wheel, parts 1 and 2, and continue with your mirroring exercises!
- Continue your *High Octane Diet*
- Continue your exercise regime... but this week add in one extra 30-minute workout, and one more gentle walk! You should now be up to three, 30-minute workouts per week and three gentle walks. Remember to do your affirmations on your walks too! And keep doing your V-12 Turbo Boosts five days/week.
- Weigh in daily or weekly and track your changes.
- Drink 8-10 cups of water each day

Week 6

Slow Down; Read The Signs!

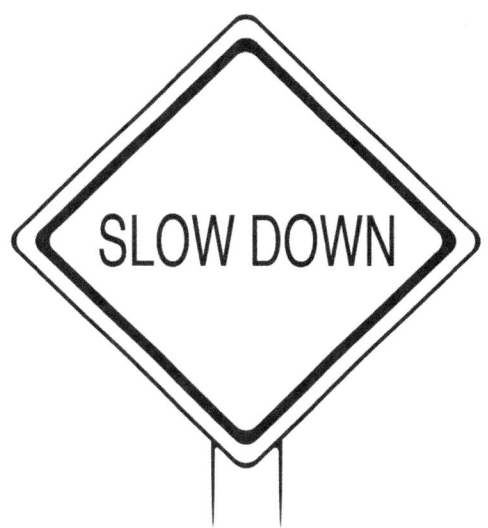

Have you ever been traveling, jumped on a new freeway, and five miles down the road realized that you hadn't been paying attention to the speed limit signs? *Is it still 65 MPH here, or did they lower it to 55?* Panic sets in and you imagine what you'll say to the police officer when he pulls you over. It is easy to zone out and drive mindlessly, and miss the signs altogether. Unfortunately, women often do the same thing with their bodies. One of the most important aspects to gaining a healthy mind and body, and attaining those goals on your Vixen vision board, is learning to be aware of the signals your body is giving you. Your body has it's own rhythm and voice, and when you learn to tap into it and notice when something is amiss, or even when It is going splendicly – you will be able to connect your daily habits with a corresponding consequence, and you will be better equipped to make choices that serve you. This week you'll gain the tools you need to stop, look and listen to the cues your body is telling you, and interpret what it all means.

Recently I attended an event at my son's school. He was being rewarded for maintaining a 4.0 GPA average throughout the school year (I KNOW! So proud of him.) However, when I pulled into the school parking lot, I knew I was not in the right frame of mind to support him or receive the blessing of watching him be honored. I was heavily burdened mentally and physically – I had been under a lot of stress in my professional life, and I had allowed the workload to prevent me from getting the proper amount of sleep each night. My body and mind were both overtaxed. There were things that were happening in my life that I couldn't seem to shake that night because I was so tired. So before going in to my son's event, I decided to use a gear-shifting technique to clear my mind, and re-focus on the moment. I stepped out of the car to a beautiful clear sunny day. As the breeze blew over me, I closed my eyes and took a deep breath in through my nose. I envisioned with that inhale an ocean wave cresting, and as I exhaled the breath through my lips, I imagined the wave curling over my head and breaking at the nape of my neck – dispersing all of the negative thoughts and energy. I repeated this three or four times until I felt calm and present in the sights and sounds around me, and then proceeded to go inside the building. Throughout the ceremony, if any unwanted thoughts crept in I immediately used the same tool, right where I sat, to let them go. This was a physical stress reducer (using the breath), as well as a mental (using visualization) stress relief. After about five times of catching those incoming negative thoughts, they stopped returning, and I was able to focus wholly and completely on enjoying the ceremony.

⸻

Stop

That story illustrates a good point. Sometimes we can get wrapped up in anxiety or worry, unable to separate the problems of yesterday, or the fears about tomorrow from the events of today. I have heard it said that men have compartments, and women have baskets. Men can take an unsolved problem, shelve it and deal with it tomorrow, to better focus on the current task at hand. Women, on the other hand, carry baskets into which everything is thrown. And we seem to never put the basket down either – we drag it to work or out with friends, to our child's school event, or to family game night, we haul it into our bed with our husbands, and we let that all that "stuff" interfere with our attitude, our relationships and our health. To make a change – We need to stop the mental chatter and we need to stop the chronic stress.

Human beings are wired to experience fear and anxiety, and some of it is good – it serves an evolutionary purpose, by protecting us from dangerous situations. But if you allow worry to continually assault you, you will never enjoy life because you are constantly stressed and anxious. In addition, that chronic anxiety causes insulin and cortisol levels to soar, which will lead to belly fat, which is a precursor to heart disease and other illnesses. Often, negative worrisome thoughts may keep you up at night, or disrupt your sleep – leaving you physically and emotionally exhausted. And if you don't get enough sleep, those thoughts will worsen throughout your day. So whether or not it's due to lack of sleep, when your mind is spinning with these unproductive thoughts, you need to let them go. The sooner you do, the better. To help relieve yourself of your current train of thinking, as soon as they start creeping into your head, ask yourself if its taking your attention away from something else that serves you better. I guarantee that it is. Whether it serves you better to focus on a conversation with a loved one, or it serves you better to be more productive at work, or it serves you better because you need to get a good night's sleep, negative thinking and mental "chatter" do not serve you... EVER!

Sometimes our fears and anxiety gets the best of us though. And no matter how hard we try to push those thoughts out of our minds, they just won't go. If you feel its absolutely necessary to worry or ponder on a situation, and your gear-shifters aren't working too well, then as crazy as this sounds, go ahead and block out 15 minutes of the day to fret over your concerns. Even just "knowing" that you have a time when you can think about your worries, will ease the stress. Your designated worry time could be spent taking a walk, which will allow you time to contemplate. In addition, the increased blood flow from the exercise will cause you to think more clearly and keep things in proper perspective. Or, maybe your worry space might simply be a quiet corner, or a special chair that you retreat to during that time. Whatever it is, use a tool that works for you, making space in your day as a designated time and place to sort through your problems. So when you begin to hear that mental "chatter", stop and breathe, and tell yourself, "I'm tackling these thoughts during my designated time and place". And when that time comes, just remember, that when your "worry" time is up, put those thoughts back in their compartment and walk away.

If you, like most women I know, wake up in the middle of the night and find yourself thinking of a million things and you can't get back to sleep, try a trick that I use. Don't waste time tossing and turning. As soon as you realize that you can't get those thoughts out of your head, get up and go to the kitchen and drink a glass of milk or hot decaf tea. Get out a piece of paper and write down everything on your mind. This may take up to 20 minutes, but it will save you hours of sleep deprivation. Then schedule a time the next day that you can go through that list and resolve those issues. Take a deep sigh of relief and go back to bed, knowing that it will all get taken care of tomorrow. Of course, you might want to stop by the ladies room before retiring, so that your bladder doesn't decide to wake you up in an hour! Once back in bed, as you lie there, breathe in and visualize a white light entering your body, filling it with Divine love and peace. As you exhale, blow out any unnecessary chatter that might be remaining. With your every exhale; think the word "relax" and physically feel your body melting into the sheets. Or, you can listen to a guided meditation with soothing music to help lull you back to sleep. The other thing you can do is pray and ask your Higher Power to take away those unwanted thoughts, and repeat the mantra, "I let go of thoughts, and trust that I am taken care of". Think of yourself as a baby in your Divine Mother's arms and she's rocking you to sleep, and you are completely safe. Trust in that security, and you can let everything else go.

Now, when the stress is really huge, or you find it to be chronic, with no end in sight, start using the Gratitude Wheel part 1; thinking of all the things you are truly grateful for in your life now until you actually feel that sense of gratitude. Also, as mentioned before, take deep, relaxed breaths. Begin to pay attention to what each of your senses are experiencing, and really hone in on each of them, individually; what you are physically feeling as your skin touches the surface you are sitting on, what you smell, see, taste and hear. Getting into the state of gratitude or sensually living in the present moment will bring peace to your mind and heart.

LOOK

The discipline of *looking* into yourself refers back to those triggers you uncovered at Mile Marker 4. But that is not all there is to it. Catching yourself before you go for the bag of chips to consider what thoughts were in your mind, or what circumstances you have been in today, are a large component of understanding yourself and your motivations. However real *looking* also goes deeper than that, mining your subconscious fears, as the true motivation for many of your thoughts and behaviors. While it is important to acknowledge that an argument with your spouse may be the trigger that ignites your emotions, which then drive you to overeat; it is even more important, long term, to look into the face of the real culprit that pulled your trigger – FEAR.

Perhaps an example will illustrate this best. Bev and Mark have been married now for six months, and they fight more than the average couple. They disagree about many things – what color to paint the kitchen, what movie to watch, or whether they should lease or buy their next car. But Mark loves Bev deeply, and reaffirms this daily. They both just happen to be very opinionated, and they always make up or compromise in the end. Mark feels okay about the tiffs, and is committed to Bev. But Bev sees things differently. She is also deeply committed to Mark, plans to honor her vows and stay with him forever. But, whenever they fight, she can't help but worry uncontrollably and that worry drives her to the pantry. She has gained 15 lbs in the 6 months they've been married. She acknowledges that fighting with her husband causes her to emotionally overeat. But what she doesn't understand is the deeper fears behind it. The real reason she is filled with anxiety and runs to the cupboard for comfort, is not due to the act of fighting itself, it is her deep seated fear of being rejected or abandoned. And if Bev really dug in, she'd discover that her fear of rejection drives many of her choices in life. She lives to be a pleaser – to over-commit her time, so no one is let down. She spends too much money buying lunch and gifts for friends, and she puts in more than her share at work. In fact, if Bev took our core values test, she may have chosen "acceptance" as her highest core value. Her deepest desire is for people to welcome her in, just as she is. And when she fears she will receive the opposite – she eats.

Your fears may be causing the same set of problems for you. They may be the real reason you are driven to overeat as a means of escaping present circumstances. Maybe your highest core value was "peace" and you had a verbally abusive youth. In that case you may be triggered to overeat by arguments or loud noises. Or, maybe you completely avoid conflict by not speaking up for yourself or for your beliefs because deep down you fear being yelled at or being criticized. And ironically, that same fear has led you to criticize your own appearance and self-worth. So, when you get in an argument with your husband, rather than speaking up, you clam up and hold it in, causing emotional duress, and you grab the ice-cream container and a spoon and go into your bedroom and dive in. Or, also in this case, when looking into the mirror and seeing your imperfections, you criticize yourself. You may not immediately run to the cookie jar, but perhaps later that day when the girls invite you out to lunch you find yourself overindulging in comfort foods. Looking involves more than just examining your life circumstance, it involves examining your inner woman, and being honest with yourself. Now, some of these examples may seem a little extreme to you. Or, perhaps you can relate to them. Whichever it is, as you can see by these examples, if you can eliminate the fear, you can eliminate the string of events that ultimately cause you to feel miserable and gain weight. But, how do you eliminate those fears? You must face them!

The next time you feel driven to the fridge I want you to ask yourself the questions from Week 4 to determine your triggers, thoughts, emotions and fears. Once you identify your fears, then take some time when you are alone and its quiet and you can relax, breathe deeply. Take out your journal and look at your list of fears. Look at one fear at a time, and don't overdo it by exploring too much at once. Relax, breathe deeply, and close your eyes and imagine that fear coming true. What would you do, how would you feel? Allow yourself to live in *that* moment of believing that your fear had come to fruition. Just like you visualized your beautiful future you… I want you to visualize your greatest fears. This could be painful, and it may bring tears - but do it, relaxing through the whole thing, just breathing. What would you do if it were true? Where would you go? Who would you call? Is it life or death? What if it is? Then what? Many times when you face your fears, you'll discover that they weren't really as bad as what you thought. And sometimes they are, but then you move on. One of my greatest fears while I was dating Brett was that I would lose him. My greatest fear came true. Was it horrible? Yes. Did I survive? Yes. And not only did I survive, the year after his death was life changing for me. What I discovered is that I had nothing else to fear, because I had experienced my greatest fear and it helped me to live life more fully, knowing that no matter what, I will be okay.

Fear robs you of personal power, and drives you to make unhealthy choices. If this process seems too overwhelming for you to imagine, I encourage you to get someone to help you with the process if needed for direction and perspective, whether that be a good coach or a therapist. Having someone to talk to will also help draw out inner truths that you could not reach on your own. For more information on getting coaching, go to: www.vixenunleashed.com.

In addition, just by being focused and aware, you can prepare yourself in advance for situations that typically cause you to eat in excess. For example, if preparing to have a difficult conversation that you know might spark a little tension and uneasiness, be prepared. Have a cup of hot tea and do some meditation prior to sitting down to talk. And also know what your gear-shifter will be if something springs on you that takes you by surprise! If you are always on the Lookout, watching for those triggers, a pattern will form. You'll know when to expect them and how to be prepared, whether it be with deep breaths, mantras, healthy snacks or you favorite gear-shifter tool. Be careful to stay on the lookout for emotions, thoughts and circumstances that threaten to run you off the road.

LISTEN

The sensations you feel in your own body are the best feedback tool you can receive about what habits and choices work and what don't. Too many women go through life detached and disconnected from their own bodies - barely registering that they pop a few ibuprofen each morning for a chronic headache, hardly noticing how many hours of sleep they got or whether they remembered to take their supplements that day. But, your body will communicate with you, for bad or good. Perhaps as you've traveled down Interstate Vixen12, you've noticed how good you feel physically. Are you more energetic, less groggy in the afternoon? Do you sleep better at night? Are the stomachaches that used to plague you a thing of the past? What if you took a "day off" from the program and had a candy bar? I bet you remember how that felt! Did you have a headache, a sugar buzz, the subsequent crash and sugar-hangover the next day? If you have, it was shocking wasn't it?

Something similar happened to me not so long ago... It was "Spirit Night" for my son's football team at a local restaurant. I went out with my family and decided to eat a half of a hamburger (with the bun) and a cola. I knew it wasn't the healthiest choice for me, but I didn't dwell on my decision, or beat myself up for doing it. I just decided that I would eat the burger and cola in moderation. After months of not eating sugar and wheat, I am sure you can guess what happened – the headache from the sugar was instant, and my stomach was immediately sick. My body clearly didn't want the cola and burger, and I knew that when I had it. But it was a decision I made at the time, and because of my physical reaction to the food, it's a decision I probably won't make anytime in the near future.

You should be taking the time each day to check in with your body, and listen to what it is telling you. When you wake up in the morning, are you refreshed and well rested? If you are groggy, you need more sleep and should plan to go to bed earlier. Are you stiff or sore? Set aside a few minutes to march in place to warm your body up and then do some long deep stretches to get the blood flowing. Midday do you have a headache? Perhaps it's caffeine withdrawal, that piece of candy you grabbed from your co-worker's desk, or dehydration. When was the last time you visited the restroom – are you sure you're drinking enough? Maybe your stomach feels overly full, you are bloated, or your weight was up. What did you eat the day prior? Maybe the issue is hormonal. What about your mood – are you grumpy, or edgy or is your mood swinging wildly? Perhaps it is something you ate that does not agree with you – sugar and processed carbohydrates actually have a dramatic effect on mood, or again – maybe you are over tired or stressed. These are a few examples of physical maladies, and possible explanations, but there are many more I didn't name. It is important to listen to all of these signals your body is giving you that something is amiss. In addition, it is equally as important to listen to the *good* feedback your body gives.

When you feel light and energetic, focused, calm – make a note of these times. What lifestyle choices have you been making that lead to this sense of well being? Perhaps it is the healthy diet, coupled with a great night of rest, the walk with your neighbor and the meditation you practiced this morning. If you know what makes you feel good you can replicate that to keep the momentum going, or use it as a remedy when you are not feeling your best.

Journaling about all of this feedback will help you pinpoint what is going on, and if you are a visual learner, reading it back will help it stick. Either way, being able to compare the headache you had last month with the one you had today can be invaluable. For example, let's say last month you had a powerful headache after work and documented it in your journal when you got home. In your journal you wrote: "Up early today when the smoke alarm went off, couldn't get back to bed. Did yoga DVD before work. Ate usual diet, drank enough, had 1 coffee, and 2 tiny bites of birthday cake at work for Sarah's party. Got in confrontation with boss before coming home." And you compare that to today's entry: "Dog woke me up at ten after four this morning, barking when our motion detector lights went on. Went for a longer walk than normal since I had the time. Diet same, no coffee for last 2 weeks. All quiet at work, but traffic was nightmare and really stressed to get home on time to start dinner." Now, if you only read example one you could blame the headache on the work problems, the cake, or early wake up call. If you only read the second example you could blame the headache on the lack of caffeine, early wake up, or stress of traffic. But comparing the 2 side by side shows the one thread that links them – sleep. It seems that if our example woman doesn't get enough sleep or is awakened mid-sleep cycle, she will inevitably develop a headache. She can remedy this by going to bed a bit earlier those nights and by being extra kind to herself. Now she knows how important sleep is for her body. Now she can listen when she gets a headache and know the reason may well be that she is just tired. You can practice the same form of listening in your own life, and it is absolutely essential that you do! By doing this, you are actually practicing becoming more *aware*.

Remember, by taking the time to STOP and be aware of thoughts that aren't serving you, LOOK deeply at all of your possible emotional and physical triggers and LISTEN to the feedback your body is giving you at every moment, you can take better care of your overall health and navigate your journey with more confidence. One of the most beautiful things a woman can be is in touch with herself, and living in harmony with the rhythm and requests of her body. Once you are doing this, you will no longer be on the physical and mental roller coaster of guilt and shame associated with avoidance, binge eating and fear. And now that you are halfway to Freedom, next week you'll learn how a new coat of paint can make all the difference in your confidence, and allow you to drive steadily towards your dreams!

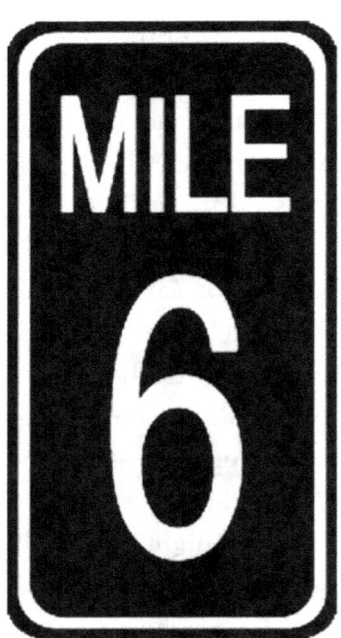

Action Steps

- Develop a list in your journal of gear shifting techniques that you can use to drive away any mental chatter or negative thinking that doesn't serve you.
- Journal about any known fears. Practice "facing" your fears and write down any thoughts or feelings you experienced. Contact me if you feel like you want a good coach to help you through this.
- Make a point to check in with your body throughout the day, and complete a head to toe sensations check. Is there anything that feels out of place or off?
- Continue to work parts 1 & 2 of the Gratitude Wheel and your mirroring exercises
- Continue with the *High Octane Diet*
- Continue your exercise regime… including three, 30-minute workouts, and three gentle walks! Remember to do your affirmations on your walks too! And don't forget your V12 Turbo Boost exercises, five days per week.
- Weigh in daily or weekly and track your changes.
- Drink 8-10 cups of water each day

Get A New Paint Job.

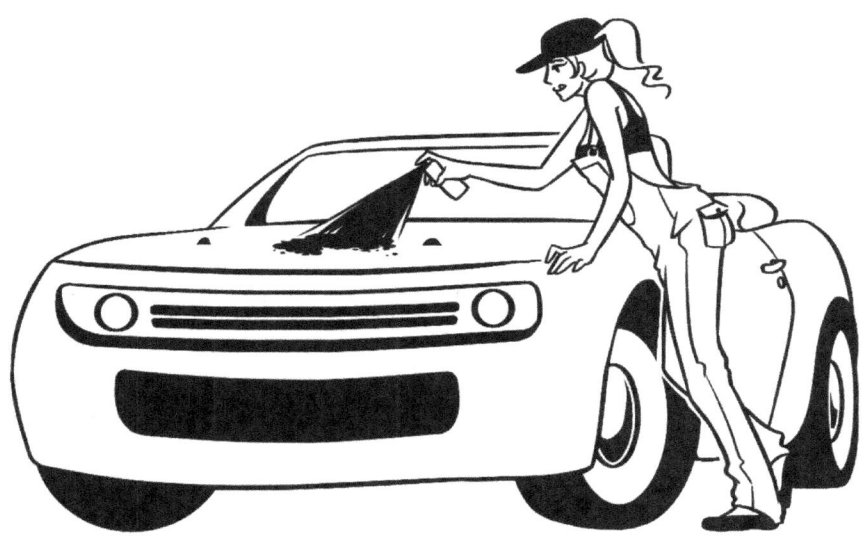

Have you ever seen a classic car that has had better days? It's rusted out, with fading paint, missing wheel covers, a dented fender? It doesn't matter how well it runs, or plush the interior is – if it looks a wreck on the outside, it is hard to be impressed by it. What that car really needs is a new coat of paint, so that the meticulous restoration that was done on the inside will shine through on the outside. This week you will be getting a new coat of paint yourself, by performing a wardrobe makeover, to better reflect all of the hard work you've done so far. You'll also set a vision for the new lifestyle you are going to lead as a Vixen Unleashed, as well as learn how to transform right now by faking it 'til you make it!

I still have the Vixen vision board I created years ago, and I refer to it often. Interestingly, what I see in my mind's eye as I think on my Board now, is not the positive phrases and photos of my future self, but it is the actions and activities I longed to take part in. You see, for me, being a Vixen was about a level of freedom I never knew, a body and attitude I'd always longed for, but most importantly — it was about being a strong woman who was confident, stood her ground and spoke what was on her mind. I had always been a peacekeeper, as many women are prone to be. But when I created my Vixen Vision Board, the most important component was to be bold and strong, to have no fear of expressing my true self, like many of the women I admired. Recently I had a difficult conversation with somebody, and was challenged in a way that would have made me shrink back and keep quiet in the past. But instead, with much maturity, I stood my ground and argued my case. I didn't allow myself to be bullied. After the talk was over, I reveled in the fact that I had come so far as a woman. My body, mind and spirit all have transformed into the Vixen I had dreamed of becoming.

TRAVEL SIZED VIXEN VISION BOARD
PART 2

This week you'll be adding more to your Vixen Vision Board, as you write out what types of activities and actions you'll take part in, as a result of your life change. Naming what you will be doing when your journey to Freedom is complete will be a great motivation towards reaching your goals. When you are tempted to stray from Interstate Vixen12, you will be able to use visualization to see yourself on the beach with your family, riding a bike with your girlfriend or asserting yourself at work, to remind you of why you are on this journey. These goals you envision for yourself are not just related to your body size and energy level, but will be reflected in how you use your time, and feel about yourself. Many women who are very overweight avoid or are unable to do certain things with family or friends, such as ride amusement park rides, join a recreational sports team, go on planes or live out personal thrill seeking adventures such as sky-diving or bungee jumping. Still others, due to body confidence issues, avoid attending weddings, parties, nightclubs, beaches, public pools and the like. These restrictions you've placed on your abilities may really be physical, but their source can also be emotional. Perhaps you are truly unable to play volleyball in the evening league with your colleagues. But maybe the reason you don't join is because your mind and confidence are holding you back, not your body. When you truly unleash the Vixen who lives inside, you will begin to do things you never dreamed of doing – no matter what size you end up being. Even though you may not yet be at your goal size, your Vixen can go to the beach with pride and confidence because she has changed the way she feels about herself and views her world. Look at my example – my body size never prevented me from being bold, speaking my mind, and owning my personal truth. But my confidence did. Unleashing the Vixen within did not simply mean smaller thighs and a new wardrobe. It meant personal power and freedom for me. So, what does it mean for you?

If you are unsure of what types of things your Vixen will be doing – you can begin by listing the physical activities that you would love to take part in, but don't. Do you throw the ball to your child or grandchild twice, before you have to sit down? Were you a little fish growing up who just adored to swim, but haven't been in the water in years? Do you turn down party invites because you don't feel good in any of your clothes or are tired of comparing yourself to the other women? Well, ask yourself – would your Vixen do that? The strong and sexy woman inside that you are drawing to the surface – is she tired, frightened, shy? Of course not! So think about all of those things that your body holds you back from doing, and begin making a list of them to add to your Vision Board.

Another way to determine what activities and actions you dream of taking are to look at people you admire. Forget bodies and style – focus on characteristics. It may be helpful to revisit your Core Values test, when you named some of your personal inspirations. Is one of your heroes a peacemaker or dedicated volunteer? Is she an activist, speaker, coach, or incredible friend? Maybe she makes herself a priority by going on hiatus twice a year to spend time in a cabin alone. Perhaps you are jealous and wish you could treat yourself to that, but felt you never deserved it. But you do! So put it on your list. I have always admired my neighbor, Roseanne who volunteers her time with the children's sports teams – driving groups of kids to and from practice and volunteer activities, over seeing them like a mother hen. When she is not doing that, she is working with developmentally disabled children and raising her own family. The time she makes for volunteerism and enriching the lives of children is an inspiration to me, and something I aspire to. Is there anyone who inspires you? Think about what qualities she has and activities she participates in that you'd like to as well.

Finally a great way to decide what you'll be doing is to reflect again on your conflicts, struggles and fears. Are you frightened to speak in front of groups or swim in the ocean or go out dancing? Are you afraid to go hiking by yourself or make new friends? Would your Vixen be scared? Think on that – you are not simply freeing yourself from the burden of extra weight; you are also freeing yourself from apprehension and poor self-esteem. A Vixen isn't frightened to be who she desires to be, who she was made to be. Imagine that all obstacles are cast aside, and you can be and do what you never dared to dream of. That is who your Vixen is, and that is your motivation to see this journey through on Interstate Vixen12.

So now that you have done the work and made your list, it's time to add it to your Vision Board. On the back side of your tri-fold Vision Board (your travel brochure), using the right hand flap that folds in, write out your list of activities using present tense words and phrases such as: "I play soccer in a weekend league", "I am running for town council", "I go rock climbing", "I volunteer at a senior center".

In addition to adding to your board, I also want you to write a Vixen Vision story, in the 3rd person, starring you! If you remember I did a similar exercise years ago after Brett died when I wrote about the man I hoped to meet. It was eerie how closely my husband Todd matched the vision I authored. Use the story to write about the woman you want to be – it doesn't have to be perfect, no one is going to read it but you. But I truly believe that writing it out, and then reflecting on it daily will bring it to fruition. This concept is called the law of attraction, and it says that whatever you focus on and seek out intently will come to you. If you focus on becoming this woman, and keep that dream before your eyes, you cannot help but to become her. That dream will guide your decision making process from how to eat, when to exercise, how to dress, act, talk, and feel. Your story should be individual to you, but here is an example so you get the idea: "Once upon a time, there was a woman named Lynne. She took good care of her body, and great care of her family. She made time for herself each day by meditating, eating healthfully, and exercising vigorously. She was grateful for life's blessings and challenges, and she was strong and confident. She dreamed to be a speaker and teach women to empower themselves, and she reached her goal. She became an author and a coach, and traveled the country showing women how to change their lives for good."Your Vixen Vision Story can be shorter or longer, more or less detailed. But I want you to reflect on it daily, carve out time for it – or lull yourself to sleep with it each night, like a bedtime story. The law of attraction will come into play, and you will start making the decisions that will transform you into this woman.

LOOK FOR WEAR AND TEAR

You've come through six Mile Markers successfully and are more than halfway to Freedom. By now you have no doubt lost some weight, increased your energy and sense of well being, as well as improved your outlook and attitude. And it is high time to have some girly fun! Some of us have a routine of going through our closets every spring or fall, pulling out what we don't like or doesn't fit, and hauling the bundle off to charity. A great habit to have, but even if you are out of the habit, this week you are going to schedule an impromptu closet raid to look for wear and tear in your wardrobe. So pick a time, grab some boxes and bags, and get to work.

Go through your closet and dresser, removing anything that doesn't fit now – whether it is too big (yay!) or too small – and get rid of it. Unless it is one special piece that you dream to fit into one day, in that case remove it from the rotation and put into storage. Wearing clothes that are too tight is unflattering and makes you look bigger than your size. Wearing clothes that are too big have the same effect, of hiding your shape and hanging tent like off of your body, making you appear larger. Your Vixen should look and feel her best, and wearing around clothes that don't fit will not make you feel confident, sexy or proud. Once you've removed the ill fitting clothes, get rid of things that are unflatter-ing to your shape or complexion, clothes that are totally out of style that you know you won't wear, things you don't feel good in, or outfits that trigger bad memories. Don't laugh! Many of us hold on to an outfit for sentimental reasons, and not good ones. It is just a dress – and if you aren't going to wear it, and it only serves to remind you of your ex-boyfriend – get rid of it! Survey what's left, you may not have much, but it's okay; we'll deal with that soon.

The next step is to grab a permanent marker and change all of the tags on your clothes to reflect your goal size! I know it sounds crazy, but as women, we already know how arbitrary sizes are, don't we? Haven't you ever gone shopping and put on an outfit 2 sizes smaller than you'd usually take and it fit like a glove? You felt great didn't you? Well, the fact is that your measurements were the same; the garment was just cut big. Even though you knew that, you were still proud to be wearing a size 8 instead of a 12. Think of it this way – whatever your tag says today is the size you are – so go ahead, change all those tags to say 6 or 8, or whatever your dream size is. And when you slide the blouse off the hanger tomorrow morning, you can think: *that's right...putting on my size 6 now!*

Pick out a color

What if you got to take your old car to the body shop and choose a whole new color for it? Sounds exciting, doesn't it? Looking at the photos and paint chips and deciding on a color that is more vibrant or exciting, that will hide the scratches and scuffs and fading? Well, now that you've weeded the bad stuff out of your closet; you get to do the same for yourself. You'll need to replace some old items with new ones that reflect the improved you. It's time to envision how your Vixen will dress and accessorize. Think back on the past - is there a time when you felt great about your appearance? What did you wear, and how did you style your hair? If you loved that time in your life, and you felt proud and confident, you can design a look for yourself that reflects your former self. Of course, if it was the 1980s, you may just want to pay attention to color and shape, and rule out shoulder pads, gallons of hairspray and parachute pants. Those things didn't look good back then! How can you update that former style to make it timeless and flattering? If there was never a time when you were proud and confident about your appearance, then go through magazines or catalogs and find styles and color palettes that you are drawn to. Think about what is flattering to your body shape, hair and eye color. Not every style works for every body – each woman has her own natural shape, which neither gaining weight nor losing it, will change. Try to find a celebrity or model who has a similar shape, whether it is hourglass, bottom heavy, slim hipped, top heavy etc, there is SOMEONE famous out there who has a similar build! Think about it, both Cameron Diaz and Jennifer Lopez are the same size, but those bodies are NOT the same. What works for one, doesn't work for the other. Consider YOUR body when designing your new look. After you have jotted down a few thoughts about style, fit, and cuts that work to flatter your body, and found pictures of styles you'd like to implement, it is time to go shopping!

Since you are still losing weight, don't buy too many new pieces now that won't fit in 2 months. Buy a few basics and some accessories that you'll never outgrow. Be sure not to buy too big or too small, but for your current size. When you try on, don't get hyper focused about bumps or bulges, or try to cover them up with out-sized clothing. Be grateful - those bulges have been your catalyst for personal growth, and you should love them. Look into the mirror and focus on how the colors and styles make you feel. Go ahead and super impose that Vixen body over yours – she is you! Buy some earrings, scarves, shoes and bags in exciting colors and patterns if you dare! Maybe you are drawn to somber colors, but for too many years you have probably been hiding behind black and gray – it's time to step out and show off your hard work! Add a little splash of color or some flash to your wardrobe, you deserve to be seen!

PIN STRIPING

Now that you've listed what you will be doing, written your story, and have a good picture of your new style, it is time to BE that woman. In truth, the Vixen you've been working hard to unleash is the woman you ARE. It is time to start being her. In essence you are going to have to put into practice that old adage – fake it 'til you make it! To become her, you have to embody her, starting right now. You are going to dress like her, act like her, speak like her, and make the decisions she would make. This is the pin striping after the car has been fully refurbished – the last important detail to complete transformation. You must start behaving like the woman you've been dreaming of, because you will not simply wake up one day out of the blue and be her. The more you practice this, the faster you will become her. So go ahead – hold your head high, and shoulders back, look people in the eye, ask for what you want in life, be strong in your beliefs and proud of your inner woman. Wear the clothes she would wear. Don't turn down party invitations or hide in the house on Saturday nights. Read your Vixen Vision Story every night to reinforce who you are. Once you get this practice into a habit, and the habit becomes a lifestyle, you will watch amazed as the weight just melts away with no more struggles. You'll become the person you deserve and have longed to be; you will become the woman that you already are, deep down inside.

In the coming week you are going to explore how to use your memories, fears, and dreams for the future to motivate you towards reaching your goal and staying healthy and strong for the rest of your life.

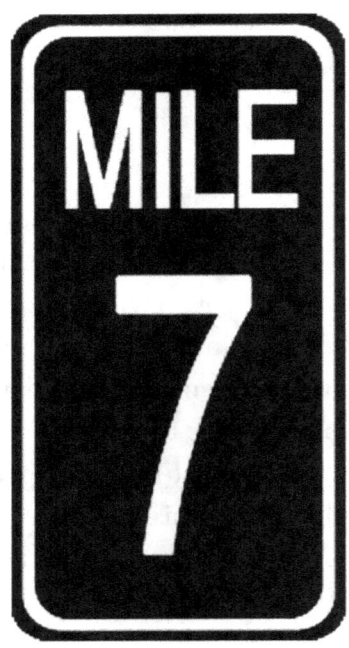

ACTION STEPS

- Complete Part 2 of your Vixen Vision Board by adding actions using present tense language to the right fold in flap
- Write your Vixen Vision story in your journal
- Take inventory of your clothes, purge the unwanted pieces, change labels to your goal size and design a new look
- Go shopping for new pieces for your Vixen to wear, step out of the box by adding splashes of color and flare
- Get out and BE your Vixen vision NOW! Go places and celebrate the new, improved YOU!
- Continue to work parts 1 & 2 of the Gratitude wheel and your mirroring exercises
- Continue following the *High Octane Diet*.
- Continue your exercise regime… including three, 30-minute workouts, and three gentle walks! Remember to do your affirmations on your walks too! And don't forget your V12 Turbo Boost exercises, five days per week.
- Weigh in daily or weekly and track your changes.
- Drink 8-10 cups of water each day

Journey With Purpose...

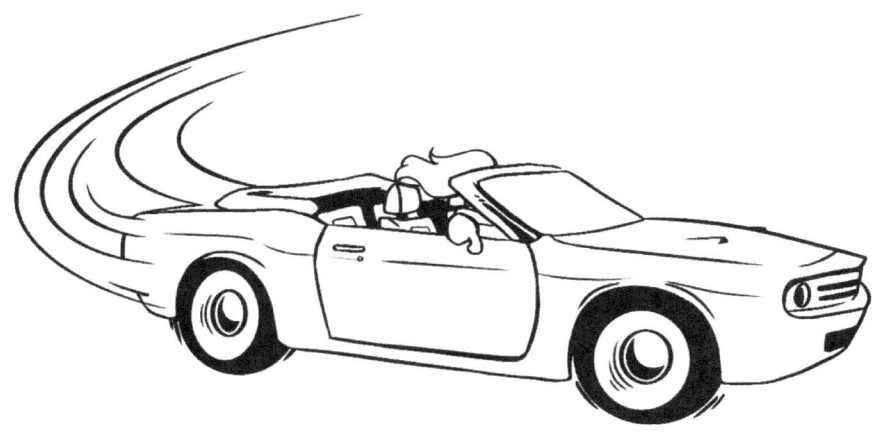

You have made great progress towards Freedom, and no doubt have uncovered a myriad of reasons to motivate you on this journey. But the best reasons to travel towards Freedom may have yet to be discovered. Once you have unlocked the true motivations for change, you can be certain they will trump any temptation or roadblock along the way. What you need now is a core reason to keep the car on the road and speeding towards your new life. This week you'll be discovering the deeper catalyst to stay with the program, learn to use painful and pleasurable memories to push you, and you'll finish up the final piece of your Vixen Vision Board.

I had many reasons to change, but my strongest reason, was the desire to be the best mother I could be. Unfortunately, I had let myself get so overweight that I simply didn't have the energy to keep up with Jake (my son), and it upset me. I began going through early stages of menopause at the young age of 36. So, not only was I overweight, I was tired, hormonal and forgetful. And because of my determination to be successful at my job, my mind was always on work and I really struggled with staying in the moment and keeping my focus on Jake. My mind would often drift back to my to-do list or catalog of anxieties. One of my core motivations to change was to be a better mom to him — to be present, and able to play with him, share and listen. If I was going to be spending most of my time at work, I wanted to ensure that the time Jake and I spent together was quality time, and that I could help instill positive values in him at an early age.

DRIVING WITH THE TOP DOWN

Years ago when I worked for the college, my work life was very demanding. Sometimes, after a day of work, on my way home I'd drive with the top down in my convertible. As I'd cruise down the road, and the wind would whip my hair around, I'd imagine all of the stress blowing right off the ends of my hair, forever lost to the wind. It was a great way to get my mind off of work. It was a powerful tool I used to let go. I have to admit, that even though it was tough, I am very grateful for that time in my life. Every day that I worked there, the stress I endured forced me to develop tools I needed to release it. Those are the very tools I use today to help my coaching clients get through challenging times! I learned a lot about my abilities and myself during my 10 years at the school. But there did finally come a day when I had to face the fact that if I constantly have to use stress-reduction tools just to survive at my job, then maybe that job was no longer right for me. Not only did I need to look inwardly to get rid of this chronic stress, I also needed to change some external factors too. That was difficult, because I was the primary breadwinner in the family at the time, and the thought of losing my income frightened me. What I really needed to kick me in the butt and make that change was a reason that was even stronger than that fear of losing my income. I needed something big to get me out of that lifestyle once and for all.

Whenever we want change in life, we will cite various reasons for making it happen. But often the reasons we give are superficial, like losing weight to look good for a class reunion, or to fit into an old dress. Perhaps those surface reasons we give are part of it, but long term, they certainly aren't enough to keep you motivated. What happens after you can zip the dress up, or wow them at the 20-year reunion? Now that the motivation is gone – will you slip back into your old ways? To make this life change truly sustainable, you have to be firmly rooted in your reasons for long-term life change. So you are going to need to dig deeper and find your most intimate and powerful core reasons for wanting a healthier mind and body.

Let's revisit that dress. Maybe it is not the garment at all that you want to physically fit into, but how fitting into it made you feel emotionally. What did you experience when you used to wear that dress? Did you feel proud, healthy, empowered? *That* is a core reason for wanting to change. The woman you want to be may possibly be someone that you once had, and then lost. Or maybe you've never experienced knowing your true self, ever! Perhaps your motivation is health concerns or fear of becoming what your mother or aunt became, living a lifetime of obesity. This can be a strong core reason as well.

Spend some time thinking about the life you've been living as an overweight person. What really scares you about the idea of staying this way? Is it chronic health problems in old age, or a pre-mature death? Is it feeling like an outcast forever? Or perhaps it's never getting to have all of the adventures you dreamed of. Or maybe your deepest fears are passing away before you get to see your kids or grandkids graduate from High School. Really think about this. And remember, these are *your* core reasons for wanting a healthier lifestyle. Only *you* can determine what they are. And again, that's going to take being honest.

In your journal list all of the reasons, big and small that you may have had — like wanting to look good for your vacation, or fit into a favorite old dress, as well as anything else you can think of that will motivate you long term, specifically things you may be afraid of, concerning your weight. For me it was the prospect of missing that precious time with my son, and not having the ability to make wonderful family memories for him. If you are having trouble thinking of anything — close your eyes and imagine yourself as an overweight elderly woman at the end of her life, who has spent most of her days being heavy. What does she regret as she looks back over her years? What did she miss out on? Those answers will give you a good indication of what it will take to keep you on the right road. Your core motivator will be individual to you, but whatever it may be, digging deeper and uncovering the reasons to change your life is essential to getting there and staying there.

PRESSING ON RAIN OR SHINE

Another great tool is to use painful and pleasurable memories or desires to motivate you on towards your goals. They both work, so learn to harness that power, and employ each of them. Though, in my experience, I think pain is sometimes a better motivation than pleasure. Once you've burned your hand on the stove, you'll always remember to be more careful. It creates a lasting memory reminding you to always use a potholder, and make sure the burner is off and cool before you set anything down on it. Similarly your painful life experiences will remind you to make better choices, so you do not experience that trauma again.

So a few years ago, when I decided to put together an arsenal of core reasons for motivation to help me to become healthy and strong, I recalled that experience from 20 years ago when I lost the part in the movie. I never again wanted to be cast aside because of my weight, so that incident was first on my list. There were other experiences that served me well when compiling this list; like when I spent a week in the hospital being observed for chest pains, or that terrible photo of myself on the beach; that became my last straw. These were all strong reasons to help propel me forward.

I have been able to harness the power of those unpleasant experiences and turn them into a new lifestyle for myself. Part of that power comes from being grateful that those experiences happened… for, without them I may not have been writing this book today. What about you? Did you watch a friend suffer miscarriage after miscarriage; while her doctor told her the infertility was weight related? Have you been a victim of taunting, teasing or rejection because of your weight? Have you had difficulty dating, pleasing your spouse, keeping up with your kids, or been ostracized from a social group because of the excess pounds? Or maybe the pain you've experienced has solely been what you've inflicted upon yourself through negative self-image, thoughts and words. Either way, you can use the pain that these incidences caused to spur you on towards your goal. If you keep these events in your mind when you want to skip a workout or overeat, it will stop you in your tracks by causing you to remember the pain you felt. Just like the hot burner on the stove. Pain is not easy to forget, so use it to your advantage.

But don't forget that pleasure can be a powerful positive reinforcement of your goals too. If you can focus on the positive benefits of losing weight and gaining confidence, such as living longer, having more energy, being able to participate in sports or fun activities, feeling proud, getting compliments, or wearing the clothes you like, you will understand how pleasurable hope for the future will help you reach Freedom as well. Or you can also use past pleasurable experiences to motivate you – like recalling how beautiful and healthy you were on your wedding day, remembering how strong you felt the first time you were on water skis, or re-living the time you first rode a horse on the beach. Pleasure reminds you of what you are striving towards, not running from, so it is important to identify pleasurable motivations too.

It's true - into everybody's life a little rain must fall (inconvenient considering you are driving a convertible)! But you have to press on. Moving through difficult times without breaking down, binge eating or turning your back on your new lifestyle is important. When problems come, inevitably the stress and fear do as well, but that doesn't give you an excuse to quit. After moving through a rough patch you will see that it has made your will to succeed and your faith in yourself that much stronger, and you can use that memory to keep you on track for good.

Travel size Vixen vision board
Part 3

Now that you have discovered some real core motivations that will power you through this life changing journey on Interstate Vixen12, it's time to fill in the last panel (center back) of your Vixen Vision Board. Use the list you created earlier of your core motivations, as well as those past painful or pleasurable memories. On your board write positive words and phrases in the present tense to fill in the rest of this statement, "I continue eating healthy because _____", and list all of those reasons. This can be anything like "I want to look good in photos", "I want to go bowling with friends" or "I want to live to be 90." It's your board, and the more accurately you describe what is in your heart that you are traveling from or driving towards, the easier it'll be to use it to motivate you and make It happen!

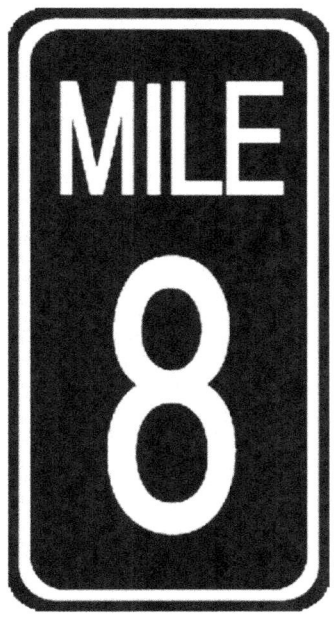

Action Steps

- Define why you want to change by reflecting on painful and pleasurable experiences, and meditating on the deeper reasons. Write your findings in your journal.
- Finish your Vixen Vision Board by identifying your core motivations to change, fill them in on the back panel.
- Continue to work parts 1 & 2 of the Gratitude Wheel and your mirroring exercises
- Continue the *High Octane Diet* plan.
- Continue your exercise regime... including three, 30-minute workouts, and three gentle walks! Remember to do your affirmations on your walks too! And don't forget your V12 Turbo Boost exercises, five days per week.
- Weigh in daily or weekly and track your changes.
- Drink 8-10 cups of water each day

Change Your Oil.

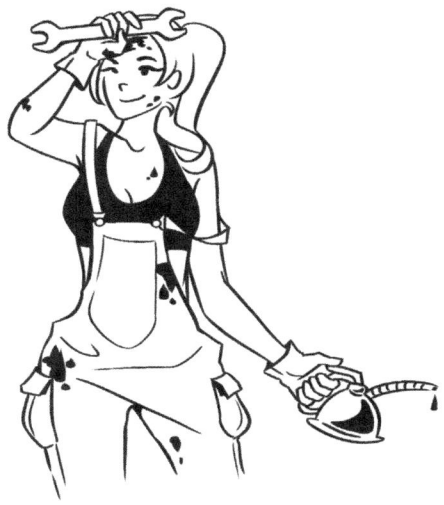

It's inevitable and cannot be avoided – no matter how much you paid for it, every car needs maintenance. You simply cannot drive 100,000 miles without rotating the tires, getting new brake pads and changing the oil every once in a while. Have you ever seen oil that has come out of an engine? It is thick, black, and may even have little chunks of debris in it. While new oil is a pale golden color, thin and translucent. What must be going on inside of that engine for that oil to come out so sullied? A better question is - what is happening inside of your brain that needs to be swapped out too?

Sometimes, despite our best efforts to relax when we are tense, or focus on gratitude instead of negativity, we just can't get there. In a hectic world where everything is demanding our attention NOW, and we are being pulled by the lure of our to do list, smart phones, gadgets and people in our lives — it seems nearly impossible to unplug, make yourself unavailable and focus on the present. This week I want to teach you the important skills of getting centered through meditation, using positive affirmations to replace the deep seated negative thoughts, and the importance of getting enough sleep to enhance your mood; focus, and lose weight more rapidly.

Recently I experienced a time when I was faced with many impending deadlines, much more than usual, and my impulse was to wake each morning and jump right into my work, rather than getting right into my workout. But one morning, instead of exercising at home I distracted myself from the temptation to work by leaving the house and all of its electronic leashes. So I woke up early, grabbed the dog and went for a run. We ended up gazing at the little pond in my neighborhood. It was so peaceful watching the ducks, listening to early morning birds without the sounds of trucks rumbling by, lawnmowers at work, or people bustling here and there. It brought me peace and relaxation that I hadn't felt in quite sometime, and it suddenly dawned on me that in all the recent busyness, I hadn't meditated in a while. I forgot to make it a priority and carve out time for it. No wonder I had been feeling stressed and overwhelmed. I vowed to add daily meditation practice back into my life, so I could short circuit the cycle of anxiety and stress.

FLUSHING OUT YOUR SYSTEM

Meditation and prayer is beneficial on many levels, and easy to accomplish. Although it really doesn't take up much time, it is still something that often goes overlooked in our lives. Truly, you need to take time out from the demands of your daily life, and making time to take care of your mind and spiritual side are as important as the time you take to brush your teeth or exercise. But we still don't do it. It is usually the brightest, noisiest, and most urgent things in life that go on top of our priority list. Forgetting to slow down and schedule the time you need to nurture your inner woman is costly, however. You end up in a cycle of anxiety, stress, busyness, and negativity. You can become resentful of the people and obligations in your life. You must make that space for yourself, and guard that time. It creates energy and positivity in you, and in turn you will have more to give to others.

One of my favorite tools to help unplug from life is using deep breathing and guided meditation. Guided meditation is simply the process of utilizing a CD, podcast, or teacher to help you relax your conscious mind, freeing it from chatter, and opening up the subconscious mind to suggestion. Guided meditation can be done anywhere that is comfortable and quiet: lying in bed each morning, sitting on the porch, or on a break at your work desk to name a few. Taking those ten minutes from your day to meditate is like hitting the refresh button on the computer – you reload and recharge. During this type of meditation you will use deep breathing techniques, and guided imagery to let go of the right now, to forget the annoyances in your life – the laundry list of problems that is always scrolling through your head. You will be talked through releasing your negative thoughts by going deep in your subconscious mind, where you are open to suggestion.

There are also other styles of meditating, even *more powerful* than guided meditation, which I highly recommend that you explore! Many people are resistant to trying to meditate on their own, without an audio guide; because they think it's too complicated or that they'll do it wrong. Or they don't want to take the time to learn how, because their minds and lives are simply too busy. If this is you, then I recommend *my* meditation guru, internationally renowned meditation teacher, and *superstar* of sensual living, Ajayan Borys. Ajayan teaches that true meditation, the deepest meditation, is not difficult at all. In fact, as he says, any form of meditation that is difficult will not be effective, because the very act of making an effort ensures the mind will stay at a superficial level of experience. Every experienced meditator knows that the best meditations are those where you just "fall into it." The trick is to be able to always fall into it, every time you sit to meditate. That's the trick that Ajayan teaches in his new book, *Effortless Mind*, which is the culmination of the 40-plus years he has dedicated to exploring and teaching meditation worldwide. The book instructs in several forms of classical meditation—chakra meditation, mantra meditation, and a meditation for health and longevity—making them readily accessible and easy to learn. So I encourage you to check it out! He covers concerns that might arise further along on your path, too, like how to fully integrate the benefits of meditation into your personality, and how to make each moment of your life a meditation. Now *that's* sensual living! To learn more about Ajayan, go to: www.vixenunleashed.com!

I know that taking care of yourself seems like a waste of time when you have so much else to do, but if you don't meet all of your needs, who will? Give time to yourself through meditation, and you will have more to give to others. Remember your Vixen Vision for yourself, it likely didn't include stressed, anxious, and pulled in 5 directions. Every modern woman needs more calm in her life – take the time to meet that need in you.

～〜

ADDING PREMIUM OIL

Meditating clears the junk from your mental engine, but to really make the motor run smoothly – you should add in premium oil by following up your meditation with positive affirmations. I love to listen to positive affirmation CDs, I have even created some for myself. I liked to time my listening to occur right after I meditated, and preferably while I was working out. Going for a run, power walk, bike ride or using a piece of gym equipment while listening to positive affirmations links your mind and body in a very powerful way. Your mind becomes more open to suggestion when your body starts moving, and naturally more receptive and positive with the release of the hormones serotonin and dopamine that accompanies exercise.

Positive affirmations force your subconscious mind to make a choice about what it is hearing. It can either resist the new truth or reappraise its current belief. For example if you tell yourself that you are worthy of being healthy and thin, you may feel a strong negative reaction to that. You will experience the resistance of that new idea and instinctively reject it at first as untrue. But the more times you hear this new thought about yourself, the sooner your subconscious will open up to the idea. Eventually, upon listening to that same affirmation, you may feel a sense of joy and well being. Your subconscious mind is beginning to accept this new truth due to repeated exposure, and your enthusiasm and passion. Gradually you will be chipping away at that resistance in yourself, and your subconscious will believe these facts and incorporate them into your psyche. Virtually every personal growth program contains some form of positive affirmations, and it is simply because they work!

Listening to your affirmations using a purchased CD or podcast from an Internet source is excellent. Or if you have the equipment, record your voice using your smart phone or computer microphone creating your own affirmations. You can also just speak them to yourself live. Write out the affirmations that you want yourself to know and believe. Look to your Vixen Vision Board for guidance. Use present tense words to affirm to yourself, who you are, such as: "I am healthy and strong", "I am courageous and passionately follow my dreams", "I experience peace in my personal life and am happy", "I love myself, I am a Divine being".

You are a Divine being. Remember your Higher Power; the Divine Feminine radiates throughout you and helps create the strong sensation that you are good; you are worthy of being loved. Your gratitude work and mirror exercises are all positive affirmations. So if you meditate each morning, I recommend that you follow your meditation with affirmations such as practicing the Gratitude Wheel and your mirror exercises to reap even more benefits, and allow those truths about yourself to sink in more deeply. Set aside the time in your schedule to include meditation and affirmations. Along with exercise, starting your day off each morning in this manner helps set you up for a dynamic and sensual day!! Of course, you have to find a time and place that is right for you – The important piece is to introduce your affirmations while you are relaxed and receptive, post meditation or prayer time.

THE PIT STOP

The importance of getting adequate sleep cannot be over stated. Lack of sleep negatively affects brain and cognitive function. Scientists have demonstrated that sleep deprivation causes delays in motor skills, impaired memory, and disrupts the healing process. [9]In addition researchers have discovered that moderate chronic sleep loss leads to weight gain and may play a role in the development of type 2 diabetes, conjecturing that habitual lack of sleep results in impaired glucose tolerance. Besides a sense of peace, energy and full functionality – sleep is important because the lack of it can slow your weight loss. Inadequate rest appears to influence your hormones by decreasing levels of leptin. Leptin is the hormone that makes you feel satisfied after you eat, which would allow you to eat more without your body triggering you to stop. Lack of sleep also stimulates ghrelin production (the hormone that triggers your stomach to rumble). [10]These two reactions combined create a perfect storm. When you are tired, to gain energy, your body is constantly triggering you to eat, but once you do, you never feel satisfied. It is a vicious cycle. Everyone has to stay up with a sick child, or go to bed late because they were traveling or working on an overdue project once in a while. But chronically disregarding your sleep needs can wreak real havoc on your health.

The healthy *High Octane Diet* you are on is a great start to the sleep equation, since you are not eating copious amounts of choco-late, sweets, or other carbs throughout the day – you are able to keep

9 Alhola, Paula; Päivi Polo-Kantola (October 2007). "Sleep deprivation: Impact on cognitive performance "

10 Taheri S, Lin L, Austin D, Young T, Mignot E (December 2004). "Short Sleep Duration Is Associated with Reduced Leptin, Elevated Ghrelin, and Increased Body Mass Index"

your hormones in check. Also, the energy you are expending in your weekly workouts and V12 Turbo Boost moves, allow you to get out your energy, sleep more restfully, and drop off easier each night. But if you have trouble sleeping, there is more you can do to ensure adequate rest. You may want to consider eliminating caffeine after 3 PM. It is also helpful to keep a journal near your bed where you can write out any worrisome thoughts that might be troubling you and keeping you awake. If you meditate and breathe deeply before turning in, you're more likely to fall to sleep faster. It is wise to limit screen time in the hour before bed, since the glow from the computer monitor or television can impair your ability to drift off. Developing a bed time routine, such as reading or listening to soothing music will set the stage and trigger you to drift away easily. Closing the blinds to fully darken your room, especially during the long days of summer, will help you control your circadian rhythms more naturally.

But how do you know if you are getting enough sleep? You should wake refreshed, not groggy and reluctant to leave bed. Doctors recommend 7-8 hours for the average adult, but everyone is different — some need more, some can get away with less. Listen to your body in the evening by keeping your awareness high. If you are beginning to feel clumsy, or spaced out, don't fight it so you can get one more thing done — go to bed! If you are getting enough hours, but still experience the problems associated with sleep deprivation, you may want to consider getting yourself checked for sleep apnea or other sleep disturbances that you may be unaware of. If you consistently have trouble falling or staying asleep, or are waking un-refreshed, consider keeping a journal of sleep habits and monitor any foods you ate that might have disagreed with you. You may want to speak to your OBGYN about having your progesterone or estrogen levels checked, you might be experiencing signs of menopause or other hormonal changes. In addition there may be something that has kept you up worrying. Writing all these potential causes of trouble down in your journal will allow you to see patterns and develop good sleep habits. Ultimately how much sleep you need is individual, and you should work towards discovering how much YOU need and be sure to get it every night. Not only will good sleep enhance your energy and mood, but also it will keep your weight loss on track by keeping your hormones on an even keel, and give you the energy you need to work out hard.

These small additions to your program truly add up to a big impact. Taking time out to do these seemingly minor tasks – meditating, using positive affirmations, and getting those extra moments of sleep, can push you over the edge from surviving to thriving. Continue to place a high priority on yourself so you can travel smoothly down the road towards Freedom!

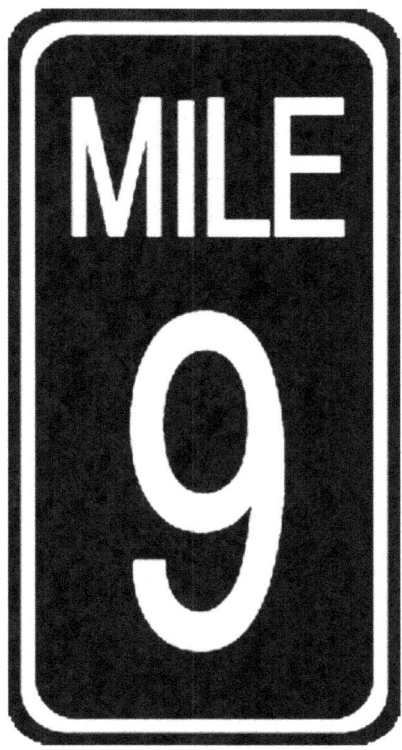

ACTION STEPS

- Add one ten-minute meditation session to your day. For resources, visit www.vixenunleashed.com
- Incorporate positive affirmations into your program for 5-10 minutes twice per day
- Get adequate sleep every night this week. Make a note of how it makes you feel.
- Continue working parts 1 & 2 of the Gratitude Wheel and your mirroring exercises
- Continue with your *High Octane Diet*
- Continue your exercise regime. But this week add in one more exercise session so you're now completing four, 30-minute workouts, and three gentle walks each week! Remember to do your affirmations on your walks too! And don't forget your V12 Turbo Boost exercises, five days per week.
- Weigh in daily or weekly and track your changes.
- Drink 8-10 cups of water each day

Week 10

Rev Your Engine!

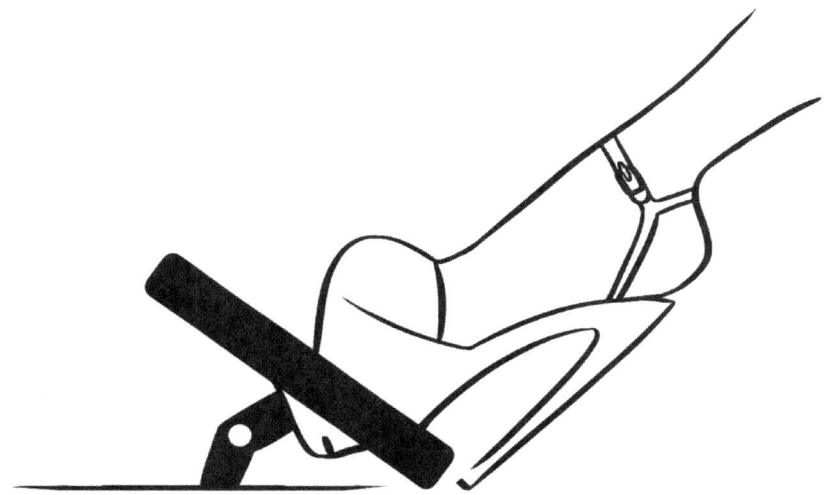

By now you are well passed the initial soreness your workouts caused and experiencing the benefits of more energy, better sleep and concentration, and higher self-esteem and body awareness. But your exercise program, just like anything in life, can grow stagnant if left unchallenged. This week you are going to be learning how to take your workouts to the next level by stepping it up! You'll also learn about various forms of exercise and how to incorporate the ones that are right for YOU into your life. And you'll discover how deep breathing techniques can increase your metabolism to blast fat off faster.

Once, not so long ago I was craving something different for our family time. We talked it over and decided to go for a bike ride at a nearby beach. Now, I have to be honest, I have a bicycle but it is not my favorite form of exercise! But I wanted to be with my family and decided that I was far too stuck in my routine, so I pushed out of my comfort zone, knowing it would be great family time. And you know what? I had a blast. It was a wonderful experience going out and enjoying nature together, and my thighs got a heck of a workout pedaling over the causeway bridge! It showed me that I was stuck in a rut with my exercise routine, and I set a new challenge for myself to mix up my workouts more and continue to try new things.

INCREASE YOUR SPEED

Being in a comfortable rhythm serves you because you can depend on getting the exercise you need. But it is not good to always do the same things the same way. To keep your body and mind interested and excited, and to break a plateau in weight loss or fitness level, you have to change things around. Now is the time to really make the effort to go for it – upping the duration of your workouts, increasing the incline, resistance or speed on the cardio machine, or trying new forms of exercise. This week I encourage you to look into new programs and forms of exercise to see what might interest you. Perhaps it will be something that scares you, or that you've always wanted to try but never quite had the courage. Sometimes where you think there is a physical barrier, you are actually experiencing an emotional or fear based one – like worrying how you look in your workout clothes, fearing you can't run because it'll lead to joint pain, going to the gym and putting yourself "on display", or avoiding yoga because you are not coordinated. Many times those thoughts are simply fears that replay again and again in your mind. So ask yourself: is my future self, the one I am striving towards, afraid of yoga pants, or falling off a bicycle? I highly doubt your Vixen Vision included fear and embarrassment. Trust me, EVERYBODY started somewhere, and even the thinnest, most confident woman was nervous and worried the first time she took a new class or tried a new sport. I know it can be intimidating to increase the speed (*What if I fall off the back of the treadmill?*) or try a new class (*I'll look silly!*), but part of being a Vixen Unleashed is learning to let go of those old fears and hang ups that have always held you back. It's time to kick your motor into higher gear!

<hr />

Know your engine and run it hard

There are many different types of exercise out there, and I guarantee you there is something that will suit YOUR personality perfectly. It's true! Perhaps you like the elliptical machine, but if you think that working out like a hamster on a piece of gym equipment sounds like purgatory, then don't fret, because there is an activity out there that you can do to break a sweat and enjoy yourself! With the variety of indoor, outdoor and sports activities available, there are endless possibilities. And if you truly find something that you love, exercise will not be a chore, but a joy. Afterwards, we'll go over some of the benefits that strength training, cardio, and flexibility workouts, can provide for you.

To really find out what is the best activity for you — it is helpful do to a little investigating into your personality. Are you a lone wolf, or do you like spending time with friends? Are you outgoing or shy? Do you enjoy the outdoors or struggle with distaste for bugs and weather? Are you competitive with yourself or against others? Do you like your workout time to calm you and bring a sense of relaxation and centeredness, or invigorate you and get you excited for your day? Depending on your answers, you will be able to identify many activities to try. As I see it, there are four different categories of exercise. Read through the descriptions below and see if anything jumps out at you or appeals to you more than the others. I encourage you to try something from each group to see if they are a fit for you.

Group fitness is great for social butterflies. If you love to get together with girlfriends, talk, laugh, and have fun — classes may be for you. Within this category there is such a wide variety that it's mind boggling, and you'll find something to do even if you have no rhythm. If you like riding a bike or being in the water, you'll find spinning, group swim classes or water aerobics will give you the fun social activity you crave and the great workout you need. Group aerobics classes or belly dancing will get you moving to good music and sweating alongside your friends. But don't think of traditional gyms as your only source of group fitness — what about a ropes course at a rock climbing gym? Or try a hip-hop or ballroom dance class? Acrobatics and aerial arts are also hot new fitness crazes where you'll be sure to laugh a lot and have a great time while tumbling and twirling! Have little ones? There are mommy and me yoga and stroller jogging meet-ups in every major city. Be creative, involve a friend, and experiment until you are having a blast, while blasting the fat.

Competitive fitness is a great outlet for those of you who can't help but push the pedal down at a green light and race the sedan next to you! Everyone is a little competitive, but some of us take it to an art form. If that describes you, harness that drive and use it to your benefit. The great thing about competitive fitness is the awesome mental and emotional feedback you'll receive as you progress. By it's very nature, competing will have you continually improving by trying to go faster, harder, or longer so that you can beat your own expectations or someone else. You can train for speed walking or running races, duathlons, triathlons, or bike races. If you like water, consider swimming or crewing. Up for a good fight or gaining mega strength? Then how about martial arts, power lifting, or boxing. Like the outdoors and problem solving? Try orienteering – most cities have a club that hosts timed races to locate fixed points using map and compass skills. The great thing about these sports is that there is always a new level to reach – a new distance to try or time to break, and you will stay energized and get hooked on the sense of pride and accomplishment you feel in obtaining a new belt in karate or setting a personal record in the 10k.

If you love being outside, then outdoor fitness is for you. If you live near water you can kayak, windsurf, row or swim. If you love the peace and loneliness of the woods you can hike, climb, mountain bike, trail run, backpack, boulder, snow shoe or cross country ski. Just like being outdoors or on the boardwalk? Try roller blading, jogging, power walking, beach running or bike riding. Are you sporty? Join a soccer, beach volleyball, or weekend softball league. When you are outdoors you can free your mind from the distractions of modern society – it's electronics and constant demands. You will be able to move through your environment in a very intimate way, clear your mind and reconnect with your primal roots. You can be challenged and experience the peace and blessing of nature at the same time. There is no more sure fire way to be alone with your thoughts, heart beat, and breath than to leave the cell phone at home and go off onto the local hiking trails, with no distractions except squirrels flitting in the underbrush and birds calling to one another in the distance.

The final exercise group is mind-body fitness. These disciplines are especially good for people who need help shutting off their minds, their stress and anxiety, or have issues with focus. Yoga, Pilates, tai chi and martial arts fall into this category. They demand that you be disciplined, calm of mind, and focused on the here and now, and the precision of your movements. In yoga for example, you have to be focused on your breath and the present moment. If you are an avoider, (this describes many binge eaters and overeaters, who have a history of avoiding problems through the distraction of food) yoga will be an ultimate challenge for you. Nothing holds up the mirror of truth, reflecting your current mental reality like doing a heated Vinyasa yoga class. Don't let that scare you; it is an opportunity to grow physically and emotionally. These workouts may make you sweat, but they also bring you inner peace and calm, and utter relaxation when you are through.

If you notice – within each of these categories, there is some overlap. This is where knowing your personality and preferences comes in handy. Let's take biking for example – if you are social, but not outdoorsy, take a spinning class. If you are outdoorsy, but like to be alone – try mountain biking. If you are competitive, try bike racing or duathlons. Or let's say that you are social, want to feed your mind and body, and love nature – look for a tai-chi class happening in a local park. What if you like to be inside and love to dance, but don't want to be part of a large group – try private ballroom dance lessons with your partner, or maybe play one of those dance video games! If you have kids, this is not only a great way to get exercise, but to bond with your kids too. Change the way you think about exercise – it does not have to feel like punishment or work to be effective. Yes, you'll sweat and your body will work hard, but if you are enjoying yourself, you won't mind breaking a sweat and you'll look forward to working out.

Within these categories of exercise you will find 3 basic groupings, though many of them have cross over benefits. Cardiovascular exercise gets your heart pumping and revs your metabolism. Strength training creates lean strong muscles. And flexibility training increases range of motion and helps to protect joints and enhances mobility. All three are important, and for the next few weeks I want you to focus on getting exercise from each of these three categories.

Strength training, such as can be found in weight lifting, calisthenics, crossfit, and plyometrics is hugely important. Scientists say that for every decade you are over 30, you lose up to 5 lbs of muscle mass! The only way to prevent this is to perform resistance exercises. Why should you care? Muscle takes more energy than fat to support, so even though you may not burn as many calories in weight training, as you do in cardio exercise, you will continue burning calories after your workout is done, and throughout your entire day! It also takes up less space, meaning a 150 lb muscular woman will wear smaller clothes than 150 lb unfit woman. It also increases your bone mass, which can help to prevent the onset of osteoporosis, which is a concern for aging women. In addition, it is the only non-surgical way to change your SHAPE – increasing definition, and creating firm curves where there were none before.

Cardiovascular exercise gets your heart pumping faster, ramps up your metabolism, and prolongs your life. You will burn more calories during an hour of cardio, than you will in an hour of weight lifting or stretching. It is the backbone of exercising for weight loss, and 4 out of 5 of your weekly workouts should center on getting your heart rate up with cardiovascular exercise. In addition, every time you do your Turbo-Boost moves you are getting a fast blast of cardio that packs a double punch. High intensity interval training, such as found in your Turbo-Boost routine, has been shown to burn fat more effectively, improve athletic performance, increase your resting metabolic rate, reduce that unhealthy belly fat and even improve glucose tolerance. [11]So in other

---

11 Tabata I, Nishimura K, Kouzaki M, *et al.* (1996). "Effects of moderate-intensity endurance and high-intensity intermittent training on anaerobic capacity

words – if you want to lose weight and gain health and endurance – keep doing your Turbo-Boost moves. But if you have grown bored, I suggest switching things up – sprint up and down stairs, run, use your exercise bike, or stair stepper. Whatever you can use to get your heart rate up. And then, of course bring it back down to your level 2 intensity.

Flexibility is a key feature of a healthy body and joints and can be obtained through exercises like yoga, Pilates and dance. Flexibility training will lengthen soft tissue and increase range of motion, which helps prevent injuries. People with chronic back and joint pain often find that the benefits of yoga or Pilates stretch beyond fitness and into pain relief, reducing inflammation and realigning your spine. But that is not all – it also releases tension and researchers have found it improves cognitive abilities. [12] You should follow a basic stretching regime after each workout to delay or prevent muscle soreness.

It sounds daunting, doesn't it? Trying to get all these various workouts in – but it doesn't have to be, because many forms of exercise have benefits that span the three types. Take swimming for example – it is a great resistance workout, as well as

---

and VO2max". Tremblay A, Simoneau JA, Bouchard C (1994). "Impact of exercise intensity on body fatness and skeletal muscle metabolism". Esfarjani F, Laursen PB (2007). "Manipulating high-intensity interval training: effects on VO2max, the lactate threshold and 3000 m running performance in moderately trained males" Babraj J, Vollaard N, Keast C, Guppy F, Cottrell Timmons J (2009). "Extremely short duration high intensity interval training substantially improves insulin action in young healthy males" McDonald, Lyle. "Steady State vs. Interval Training"

12 Tilbrook HE, Cox H, Hewitt CE, et al. Yoga for chronic low back pain: a randomized trial. Kiecolt-Glaser JK, Christian L, Preston H, et al. - Department of Psychiatry, Institute for Behavioral Medicine Research, The Ohio State University College of Medicine, Columbus, OH http://www.ncbi.nlm.nih.gov/pubmed/20064902 Ross A, Thomas S. – School of Nursing, University of Maryland http://www.ncbi.nlm.nih.gov/pubmed/20105062

cardiovascular exercise. In addition, swimming is wonderful for women who have joint issues or chronic pain. Yoga is one of my favorite exercises — it forces you to focus on breath and stay in the moment. It is an incredible flexibility and strength workout, and if you practice Vinyasa or heated Bikram Yoga, you will also be getting a heart pumping cardio routine as well. At the end of class you will leave feeling relaxed and refreshed, as it is a great stress reliever to boot. In addition, yoga is fully customizable, so you need not fear about your current fitness level, sense of balance or flexibility. In yoga, you are encouraged to work to YOUR potential, and not keep up with what everyone else is doing. Other workouts such as bike riding, and mountain climbing provide you with lower body resistance training and cardiovascular fitness, where as activities such as crewing and boxing will target the upper body and give you the cardio workout you need as well.

Trying all of these forms of exercise need not be expensive — many, such as running, hiking and power walking, are free. If you aren't sure you'll like biking, borrow a friend's wheels to take for a spin. Many gyms will let you visit with a friend or on a guest pass to check out classes as well. To try a new routine for free — search the web for free videos, or visit your local library where you can borrow workout DVDs for nothing. Instead of running out and buying a huge piece of equipment, consider buying a simple yoga mat, and a set of exercise bands — you can do virtually anything and build the body you've always wanted if you creatively combine those with stretching and calisthenics.

FEEL THE WIND IN YOUR HAIR

You know that exercise is good for your heart, lungs and waistline. But how does it affect your brain, and emotions? Researchers have determined that due to the release of dopamine as a result of exercising, it is good for your mood as well! Dopamine is a neurotransmitter released in the "reward" center of the brain. It is associated with pleasant feelings and outlook. It is the primary brain chemical involved in nearly every addiction from smoking, to alcohol, illegal drugs and food. [13]However, exercising provides a natural hit of dopamine. It has also been found to decrease anxiety and depression in even the chronically depressed or unnaturally fearful individual. [14]

Getting exercise will increase your sense of well-being and give you joy and a zest for life. Remember back when you sat around at the end of the day, and didn't pay much attention to moving your body? Don't you feel so much more energetic, happy and lively now? I know it is counterintuitive, but exercise gives you MORE energy, not less. It is important to stick with those workouts and make the most of whatever time you have to get them in. Even if you have to sacrifice another activity, like keeping up with your favorite TV show, or scrubbing the dishes before bed, it is worth it to keep yourself moving, considering what it does for your body, mind and self-esteem.

When life takes an unpleasant or busy direction, it is often hard to fit exercise in. But that is exactly when it is needed the most. Just like your meditations, taking the time out to exercise will relax you, get you centered, help you sleep better and create an overall sense of

13 Addiction Science Research and Education Center College of Pharmacy The University of Texas "Dopamine - A Sample Neurotransmitter"
14 Sparling PB, Giuffrida A, Piomelli D, Rosskopf L, Dietrich A (December 2003). "Exercise activates the endocannabinoid system"

well being and calm. If you are walking through a major storm right now, it is understandable if you feel the need to shelve your workouts, or literally don't have time for them. But focus on what you can make time for. If you have 15 minutes a day, you can get three Turbo-Boost workouts in. While sticking to your schedule is ideal, you have to accept it is not a perfect world and do what you can!

BREATHE IN FRESH AIR

Breathing provides your whole body with oxygen, and without breath you cannot survive. However, so many of us go through life taking short, shallow breaths – not maximizing the potential metabolic and relaxation benefits of breathing in deeply and steadily. Adding deep breathing exercises to your *Vixen Unleashed* program will boost your metabolism as well as get you firing on all cylinders.

If you are a chronic shallow breather, your cells may literally be starved for oxygen. As a result, scientists say, your body has no choice but to store fat. A Japanese study conducted in 2010 showed a significant amount of weight was lost in obese participants after simply breathing deeply for one month. [15]It sounds to good to be true, right? But it's not – I've employed these techniques for quite some time myself and I can tell you – they work. Studies completed by California University found that deep breathing exercises burned 140% MORE calories than riding a stationary bike for a half hour duration [16]! If

15 NCBI – PubMed "The "Senobi" breathing exercise is recommended as first line treatment for obesity." http://www.ncbi.nlm.nih.gov/pubmed/20834183

16 "Oxycise": Jill R. Johnson; 1997

you combine deep breathing with exercise – it's a powerful duo. In addition, deep breathing relieves depression and stress related disorders [17], and increases the overall capacity of the cardiovascular system. Deep breathing techniques will increase your Vo2 max, which is your maximal oxygen consumption, without exercise. Leading to greater endurance, and better blood oxygenation.

The premise of deep breathing is very straightforward – you simply need to take oxygen deeper into your lungs, and expel out all the carbon dioxide. Odds are good that right now you are simply breathing shallowly into your chest, and although it's enough to survive, it is not enough to thrive. Start by performing this simple breathing exercise three times per day for 10 repetitions. To begin your "breaths", exhale until your lungs are empty. Then, to a slow count of 5, breathe in deeply through the nose, first filling the belly, then the ribcage, followed by the lungs. Once your lungs are filled, hold your breath for 15 seconds, and then release it in the reverse order for 10 seconds, blowing all that carbon dioxide out of your lungs. Now, repeat until you've completed 10 repetitions. Performing this 3 times per day will get you in the habit of breathing more deeply as a regular course, leading to a higher metabolism, reduced stress and overall sense of well being. For more on deep breathing techniques and benefits check out a wonderful book called <u>Jumpstart Your Metabolism</u> by Pam Grout

Now that you've delved deeper into better fitness, next week you'll take a look at some more interesting facts about nutrition and we're going to possibly add some new things to your diet! Keep your engine running hard by mixing up your workouts, adding focus to your strength, endurance and flexibility, and learning to breathe deeply to provide more oxygen to those hard working muscles.

---

17 Relaxation Techniques for Health: An Introduction" <u>http://nccam.nih.gov/health/stress/relaxation.htm</u>

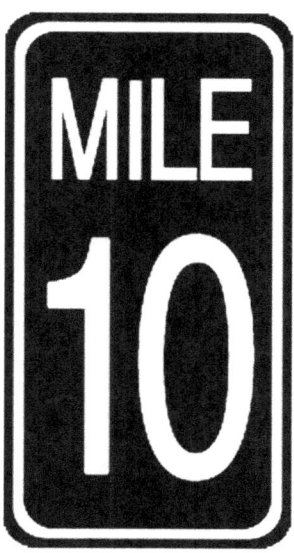

ACTION STEPS

- Try one exercise from each of the four categories this week: group fitness, mind-body, outdoor fitness and competitive fitness
- Be sure you are getting exercise from the three groups: flexibility, resistance training, and cardiovascular.
- Continue working parts 1 & 2 of the Gratitude Wheel, your mirroring exercises, and your meditation.
- Continue with the *High Octane Diet* program.
- Continue your exercise regime… including four, 30-minute workouts, and three gentle walks! Remember to do your affirmations on your walks too! And don't forget your V12 Turbo Boost exercises, five days per week.
- Weigh in daily or weekly and track your changes.
- Drink 8-10 cups of water each day

Week 11

Pumping Fuel.

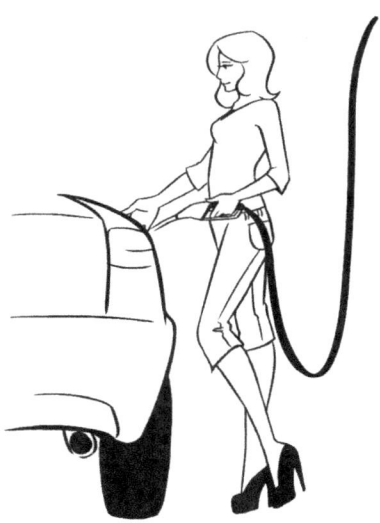

By now, you should know how it feels to fill your tank with premium, high-octane fuel. When you first started your road-trip, you began a journey that has no doubt given you fantastic results, changed your thinking about food and hopefully increased your overall sense of well being. Remember how you felt during week 1, when you moved off of the breads, gluten, sugars, and other processed foods? Maybe those first few days felt nearly impossible – like you were trying to quit smoking. Perhaps you felt pulled or called by the sweets and breads, and had to muster everything you had to stay away. And now, it's not even so much that it's easier to resist temptations, but there is a good chance that you probably don't even have the desire to eat those foods. Over the last 10 weeks, you have been doing some amazing work on your inner self, as well. You've made many positive changes in your overall health. Perhaps for the first time you feel strong, in control, hopeful and beautiful. Part of self-awareness, is knowing what your body and mind need at any given time by reading the feedback you get from your thoughts, mood, physical health, and energy levels.

If you are happy with the program, don't want for variety, and are feeling great – wonderful, I want you to stick with it just as it is. If you are nervous about the prospect of adding a small amount of gluten or processed foods into your diet and feel that you may not be able to handle it physically or emotionally – then keep everything the same for now. If however, you feel you are ready to experiment, then I will explain how to work certain items back into your diet, and test whether they are a benefit or hindrance to YOU. Every body is different, and you truly will not know how these foods affect you until you try them again. This can be an enlightening experience and I want you to journal everything you feel and witness in yourself while making these changes.

For the first week you might want to try replacing 1 grade of starch per day with whole wheat or other whole grain foods that contain gluten. Below you'll see an additional food list of starches for you to choose from that contain gluten. Try this for one week, and journal the changes in your weight, mood, energy levels, and sense of well being. Also, make sure to become aware of any bloating, headaches, bowel problems or other physical signs of gluten sensitivity. Did you experience fatigue or have trouble sleeping? Did your weight loss slow, stop or did you GAIN? After a week you should know, but even after one day – if you are not feeling well, you may realize immediately that whole wheat and/or foods with gluten are not ideal for your body, your weight loss, and optimal health. If this is the case, you should honor YOUR body and see gluten and processed carbohydrate consumption as a special occasion treat only.

Starches Containing Gluten - 1 Grade =

Breads

1 slice Bread - whole grain/wheat

1 Tortilla - whole grain/wheat (6 in.)

2 ¼ Bagel, large - whole grain/wheat

½ Bun - whole grain/wheat

½ c English muffin -whole grain/wheat

5-7 Crackers – whole grain/wheat

½ Pita - whole grain

Cereals

½ c Hot cereal (oatmeal, creamed wheat, grits, oat bran)

¾ c Cold cereal – ready to eat (high fiber, whole grain/wheat)

¼ c Muesli

Other Grains

1/3 c Couscous

1/3c Pasta, whole grain/wheat

½ c Bulgur, cooked

If and when you are feeling brave, and are strong in your commitment to yourself and your goals, I want you to think about taking ONE day to eat a few of your old favorite processed products. This would be foods like white breads or pastas, sugary treats, pastries, etc... and journal how you FEEL shortly after you've consumed them, throughout that day and the day after. I also want you to be aware of any signs of physical addiction... like once you start eating it, notice if you automatically overindulge. Journal everything...so you can look back on it to help you make future decisions about what you put into your mouth. It will probably surprise you to experience eating these foods again, and see the way they affect how you feel. I will warn you though, if your body has that real physical addiction to sugar, and you put it back into your body after 10 weeks of having none, don't be surprised if you start craving it again. If that happens, immediately go cold turkey on the sugar the next day. Read on to see what happened to me once, after going 3 months "sugar-free":

My sister drove down from North Carolina to visit my parents (who only lived about 30 minutes from me at the time). My brother had also flown into town from California around the same time. It became an impromptu family reunion. I hadn't seen either of them in a while and was really looking forward to their visit. Now keep in mind that my sister was on vacation, but she had started her new diet only a few months before, which included limiting her carbohydrate and sugar intake. One day during her visit, she and I took my mom to the ocean to get some fresh air and sunshine while enjoying the view. It was a rare occasion that the three girls in the family got to spend quality time like this together, so I soaked up every minute of it. Anyway, after a glorious and relaxing day at the ocean, we headed home to make a celebratory meal for the whole family. On our way home we saw a brand new establishment on the side f the road that specialized in Key-Lime pies (a favorite of ours). So, we stopped in to check it out. And… you guessed it. We left the new store with pie in our hands! When we got home, we found out that my brother had made a homemade key-lime pie too! Our taste buds must have all been on the same page that day! After dinner, we all engaged ourselves in a round (or two) of pie sampling! It was almost sickening sweet, but very tasty… and difficult to stop at just a little, to be honest. I cannot tell you how long it had been since I'd had sugar like that, but the shock to my body was apparent the following morning. My sister and I both woke up with headaches, totally exhausted and feeling "hung over". Throughout the day we both noticed that we also felt depressed. It was such an eye opener to introduce that food back into my diet and see how I reacted physically (headaches, low energy) *and* emotionally (depressed). To think that two little slices of pie did all that — it was mind blowing! And it was really strange because for several weeks after, I noticed myself beginning to have little bites of sweets more and more. Of course, I'm religious about weighing myself daily, and journaling my thoughts and emotional and physical feelings. So, after about two weeks of this nonsense, I made the conscious decision to go cold turkey on the sugar. Most of the time I don't eat gluten or sugar, but I do still have it occasionally in small amounts. If I start to notice it developing into a regular habit, I go cold turkey for a while. That's why it's so important to develop the awareness skills that I've been teaching you throughout this book.

Awareness of *why* you include certain nutrients into your diet for optimal health is also important. The more knowledge you have on how foods can affect YOU, the easier it is to make good decisions for yourself. For example, if I just told you to "eat this" or "eat that" because I SAY SO, you might do it because you're following a new diet book. However, if you don't understand *why* these foods are either good or potentially harmful to you, you might easily skip your veggies because they are a pain to cut up, or not buy salmon because it's too expensive. But if you are aware of the *value* of these foods in your diet, and how they can keep you healthier, live longer, feel better, and fight off cancer, etc…then you're much more likely to take the time to cut up your veggies and make that fresh salad to enjoy along with your dinner, rather than just open a can of creamed corn processed with high fructose corn-syrup. In chapter 3 you learned about the *High Octane Diet*, what to eat, how to eat, and when to eat. Dr. Keesha and I gave you that outline to help you follow a simple and nutritious plan while you worked on your inner self, began exercising more, and shed some weight. Now, I would like to elaborate a little more as to "why" certain elements of your diet are necessary for good health and energy. And we'll begin with the one of the most vital components to vitality, second only to oxygen: water.

HYDRATION

Up to 60% of the adult human body is made up of water – including 75% of your muscle tissue. Water is responsible for transporting nutrients within cells as well as taking away waste. Sometimes we may be dehydrated and not even know it. Many headaches and other minor issues can be caused by lack of hydration. [18]If you have a headache, before you grab those painkillers, instead try drinking a large glass of water, sans drugs. Give it about 20 minutes or so and see how you feel. If your headache is gone.... well then, there's your answer! You may also find it difficult to regulate your body temperature if you're dehydrated, or you might experience dry and itchy skin. It's easy to see that being in a chronic state of dehydration can lead to a general sense of malaise, and in more extreme cases, it could endanger your long term health. Being dehydrated can cause you to feel dizzy or lightheaded. Your brain will not function properly and you may feel groggy and move slowly. Your kidneys will be unable to carry away waste products, which will lead to a build up in toxins – causing you to feel ill. So, as you can see, it's important to drink enough water in order to sustain good health. I recommend at least 8 cups per day. Always carry a bottle of water with you on your errands, to and from work, or around the house. Most certainly do NOT exercise without water breaks, drinking to thirst. A simple method of testing yourself for dehydration is pinching the skin on the top of your hand. If it snaps back into place quickly, then you're

---

18 USGS – Water science school - http://ga.water.usgs.gov/edu/proper-tyyou.html

not dehydrated. If the skin goes back into place slowly, then there's a good chance you need a little H2O. The best judge as to whether you are well hydrated, is if you are urinating frequently and it is a pale straw yellow. If it is dark yellow – that is an indication you need more water. If on the other hand, it is clear – slow down the drinking or space it out more throughout the day. Water intoxication is also a real and dangerous condition so there is no need to overdo it. This is not meant to scare you… It's simply to make you aware. Now, let's talk about something a little more colorful…

PHYTONUTRIENTS

When I outlined the *High Octane Diet* for you earlier on, I mentioned the importance of eating a rainbow of colors with your fruits and veggies. Phytonutrients, or phytochemicals are an important group of nutrients necessary for healthy living. These nutrients are found in the skins of vegetables and fruits. They are the chemicals that cause the rich colors, aroma and flavors of your favorite edible plants. Colorful fruits and vegetables provide anti-oxidants and help reduce inflammation, which is a missing component of the standard American diet (SAD). There are many different classes of phytonutrients. Some classifications include flavonoids, carotenoids, polyphenols, lignans, isoflavones, indoles and anthocyanidins. Each classification has different benefits and effects. For example: carotenoids include fruits like apples and cherries and veggies like tomatoes and radishes offer immune health, prostate health, anti-cancer, and cell protection. Flavonoids are also found in the "red" category in foods such as red grape skins and red grapefruit. Polyphenols are found in "green" tea, and offer health benefits such as hormone balance and brain health, while isoflavones and lignans can be found in the "white/tan" category lentils, legumes, and soy and benefit heart health and gastrointestinal wellness. Indoles are found in foods like broccoli and other cruciferous veggies and are thought to help reduce the risk of certain cancers. You will also find foods like blueberries, which fall in the anthocyanidins category (blue/purple) that have shown benefits in weight loss in some studies. [19]

The brighter, richer, and deeper the color is in the fruit or vegetable, the more health benefits you'll get. And since they each offer something different, it's best to eat a variety, or a rainbow each day, trying to have at least one from each color group: red, blue/purple, green, white/tan, and yellow/orange. Keep this in the back of your mind when making your meal plans for the week. Again, if you are simply aware of how certain foods can benefit you, whether consciously or subconsciously, you will begin making better choices for YOU.

PROTEIN

Protein is vital for metabolism and cellular structure, forming the scaffolding that maintains the shape of our cells. Proteins are responsible for immune health, and provide amino acids, which are the very building blocks of human life. While we are able to make certain amino acids within our own bodies, we cannot make all of them! The only way to receive those all important amino acids that we do NOT make (such as Tryptophan and Leucine) is to eat them, by consuming good sources of protein. When our amino acids are out of balance we can experience nervousness, exhaustion and dizziness, or even negatively affect our long-term health. How do you ensure that you are getting enough of these all-important proteins? By following the *High Octane Diet* and having protein with every meal, of course!

19　April 20, 2009, Science Daily http://www.sciencedaily.com/releases/2009/04/090419170112.htm

Great sources of protein and amino acids are fish, chicken, lean red meat, dairy, seeds, eggs, beans and nuts. In addition, while not a major source of protein, many essential amino acids can be found in colorful vegetables, particularly leafy greens like kale and spinach. Protein supports our muscles and organs, provides a great source of energy dense calories, and does not spike blood sugar, causing the release of insulin, like carbohydrates will. Eating a protein rich meal will cause you to digest your food more slowly, leading to a prolonged sense of fullness. It is not only healthy for you, but is the perfect source of calories for the purpose of losing weight.

FAT

Nobody would argue that protein is bad for us, but what about that 3-letter word – Fat? Recently more and more doctors, scientists and researchers are uncovering that dietary fat doesn't deserve the bad wrap it once received, and in fact it is essential for good health. Fats are important for human life, serving structural and metabolic functions. They give us healthy skin and hair, insulate our organs from impact and shock, and maintain body temperature and cell function. Fat also acts as a buffer against disease – when a chemical or bacteria reaches dangerous levels in the blood stream, the body can dilute it by storing it within fat tissue – protecting our organs until the fat can be removed by excretion. Certain fatty acids are essential nutrients that our bodies cannot make, so they must be ingested. An example of these is the Omega fats – specifically Omega 3 and Omega 6 fatty acids, which are polyunsaturated fats. Proper consumption of these important compounds reduces the risk of heart disease and stroke. Getting a right balance of Omega 3 to Omega 6 may counteract or positively influence a host of health problems including depression, diabetes, rheumatoid arthritis, cancer and Alzheimers disease. [20]Unfortunately the Western diet typically is unbalanced, providing more sources of Omega 6 than Omega 3; but you can do something about this. Aim to get a 1:1 ratio of Omega 3 to Omega 6. You can get your Omega 3s from balanced fish oil capsules, fatty fishes, flax seeds, leafy greens, chia seeds, walnut oil, and olive oil. Most of us are not deficient in Omega 6, due to the high usage of soybean and corn oils in the American diet, however – if you are eating a whole food diet that is limited to mainly protein, fruits and vegetables you will want to be sure you are getting at least some Omega 6 in the form of safflower, sunflower, peanut and grape seed oils. There have been conflicting studies on the benefits of *saturated fats* such as those found in coconut oil, palm kernel oil, red meat, dairy and eggs. At the very least, saturated fat is higher in calories than other forms of fat – so you may want to use it sparingly. Though, they are not all bad due to their beneficial stearic acid content. They also contain monounsaturated oils in varying percentages, and they are much better natural sources of fat for you than using hydrogenated oil, should a recipe call for one.

Fat comes in many forms – some healthy and some not so healthy. Take trans-fats as an example. We have all heard about hydrogenated oils in the news. These are types of vegetable oils that have been chemically changed by the process of hydrogenation. Examples of these are vegetable shortening and margarine, which are created by taking vegetable fats that are naturally a liquid, and manipulating them be solid at room temperature. These fats are the exact opposite of natural or healthy – it has proven they are dangerous. [21]It's actually

20 Simopoulos AP. The importance of the ratio of omega-6/omega-3 essential fatty acids. Biomedicine & pharmacotherapy 2002; 56: 365-79 Heather Hutchins, MS, RD (10/19/2005). Logan AC (November 2004).

21 Mozaffarian D, Katan MB, Ascherio A, Stampfer MJ, Willett WC (13 April 2006).

much better for you to have a teaspoon of real butter on your veggies than a teaspoon of hydrogenated margarine.

Wow! We learned a lot in week 11. We've explored adding some gluten and possibly sugar back into our diet to see how our bodies react. We've also learned to incorporate our newly acquired skills of listening to our bodies and our emotions to see what is really best for us, as individuals. And we've learned about the importance of including lots of color in our diet, why we eat protein and fats, and why we must stay hydrated! Now it's time to move on to our final week in the program, where the rubber meets the road! But before we do, please be sure to stop at Mile Marker 11 to implement your action steps!

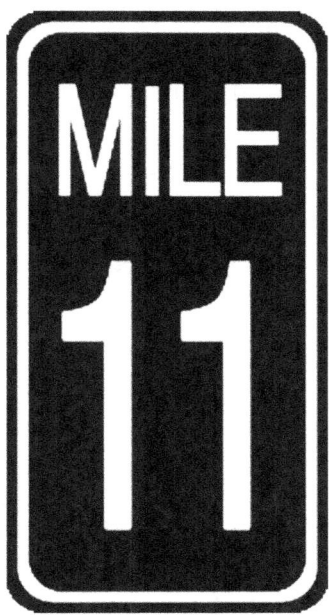

ACTION STEPS

- Experiment with adding gluten and possibly sugar back into your diet. Do it slowly and journal your physical and emotional reactions.
- Focus on getting a rainbow of color in your veggies in every day eating!
- Continue with your *High Octane Diet* plan.
- Continue your gratitude and mirroring exercises as well as your meditation.
- Continue with your exercise regime…beefing it up each week and exploring all the different types of exercises. And don't forget to keep up with your V12 Turbo Boost moves!

Week 12

Where The Rubber Meets The Road...

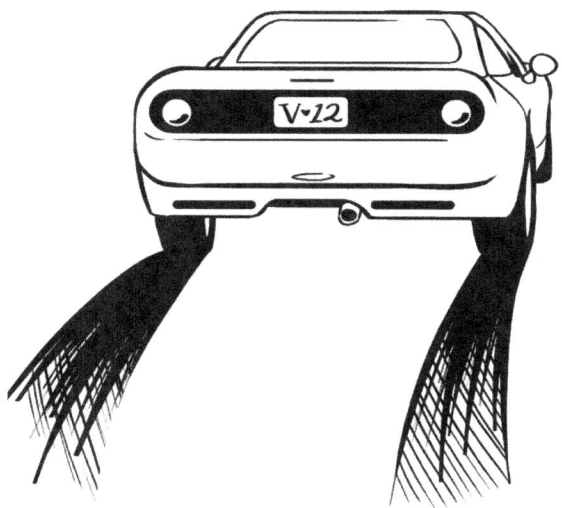

In this final week together I will show you how to create a schedule. This schedule will be your very own road map to help provide balance in your home, work and personal life. I will also be introducing the third component of the Gratitude Wheel. Here, you'll uncover new ways of viewing roadblocks and obstacles in your path, and begin to see them as opportunities for growth. And like you, I am still learning, still growing and still unleashing MY inner Vixen daily. When I notice myself struggling with something, I clear my head through meditation, then I go back and refer to my core values to help guide me.

My number one core value is "freedom". Several years ago, the mere thought of being bound to a schedule would make me cringe. For a long time I felt controlled by my job, by my responsibilities both at home and at work, and by my "schedule" that had so much packed in it, I couldn't breathe. I kept making new schedules and squeezing in more stuff. I was a high achiever, and refused to let this thing beat me! I was determined to control my schedule and control my life!!! But every schedule I made was so unrealistic, and so inflexible, that I ended up letting myself down. Needless to say, I came to HATE having a schedule! However, deep down I knew that if I wanted to get my life back, adjusting and creating a *realistic* schedule (and following it) would lead me to the freedom I desired. I had to get it out of my head that my schedule was just another thing controlling me. In other words, in order to gain control of my life... *I had to surrender the need to control*. I had to remind myself that it was simply a tool that would help me become more productive at work, and give me time for a family and personal life. So I created a schedule with a new set of priorities...and the first priority was taking care of ME! I could stay on task and in the present without the constant worry that I was forgetting something, or there was more to do elsewhere. My schedule doesn't control me – it frees me. I have found that, when I neglect to make - and follow - a proper daily routine, I get stressed, over worked and anxious. Without proper time blocked out in my planner to nurture myself, and my family, I soon become overwhelmed, run down and constantly frustrated. However, I have also learned that it's flexible. Like everything else in life... even the schedule *can change*! So... are you ready to get started? Let's go!

Creating a schedule you can live with is not difficult. Begin by turning to a fresh page in your journal, and make 6 columns. You may need more, or less depending on who and what are in your life. At the top of each column label them as follows: "Me", "Family / Spouse", "Household", "Work", "Social", "Community/ Volunteerism". You may not need every column, but then again you may have to just think more broadly about the categories. For example – if you live alone, and have no family nearby, you probably aren't free from *all* family obligations. Taking the time to call your parents once a week, or check in with your brother and his family out on the other coast, definitely fall under the "Family" category. Maybe you don't volunteer with an organization, but you watch the neighbor's children once a week so she can have a few hours to run errands. That IS volunteering! Start with those columns, but know you may need to add more. In each of them begin listing your duties and obligations. It does not matter what order they fall in, so don't fret about that now. In your "Me" column list things such as exercise, preparing your food, meditation or quiet time, journaling, reading, listening to music, haircuts, taking a long bath, etc.- anything that you do for yourself that nourishes, recharges, or maintains you. Next consider your family obligations – those to your nuclear family, and extended family. Write in playing with or reading to the kids, spending time outdoors as a family, going on dates with your spouse, visiting your parents etc. Do this exercise, thinking through a typical week or month and come up with as many of your duties as possible, even things you want to do, but have neglected.

Then, armed with your list, begin laying out your road map for the future. Using the digital calendar on your phone, your computer or a day planner, create 3 calendars: one for daily tasks, one for weekly tasks, and one for monthly tasks. For example: vacuuming is probably not a daily task, but doing the dishes or a quick de-cluttering is. Maybe scheduling a date with your spouse is not something you can do weekly, but perhaps you sneak away once or twice per month. Or maybe you decide that once a week date night isn't such a bad thing, and you add that into your weekly calendar! For my recurring daily tasks, I schedule specific times of the day to begin and end each of them – like working out, feeding my pets, showering and getting dressed and meal times. I actually use the alarm on my cell phone to remind me it is time for those things, otherwise I can get so wrapped up in what I am doing, that I'll neglect to do those basic tasks that are so important. What if you have a project you want to tackle that will take you half a day, like organizing a huge box of old photos? You don't need to wait until 6 hours magically becomes available in your schedule (which might not be until you retire!). Pick a couple of days each month, to free up for that special day to do spring cleaning, or host a garage sale, or whatever you want to do. Once it's in your schedule, you lose that "guilty" feeling of not getting ALL of your day-to-day tasks completed. Now, this is going to sound like an oxymoron, but you will have to be somewhat rigid, and you have to be flexible at the same time. If you're working on a big project, I recommend using a timer if needed so you know when to stop. Don't get so focused on that project that you go over your budgeted time, causing the rest of your plans to suffer. But also be flexible. As it gets closer to the day you had set aside to do that big project, something more pressing may have come up, and you need to allow yourself that ability to make those changes, without guilt. Always keep in mind that if it's not life or death, there is no reason to get stressed out or anxious. Just breathe, relax, and move forward. Set goals for yourself for each day, week and month, and leave wiggle room for new projects or unexpected situations that pop up.

No day planner is a respecter of emergencies, or unforeseen issues. If someone in your life (including you) gets ill or injured, that may take precedence over folding the laundry or making cookies for the school bake sale. You also shouldn't be so rigid in your scheduling that if your child asks for a heart to heart talk, or your spouse needs to vent about a work problem that you come back with – "Can't talk now, I have to mop the floor." You always need to keep in mind each and every day that you and loved ones will take precedence over the more empty tasks in life. It is all about budgeting and prioritizing your time. And just as you have to schedule work or projects, more importantly, don't forget that you should first schedule time for YOU and time with your loved ones. THOSE are the priorities on your schedule that you should be MOST rigid with!

BALANCE YOUR TIRES

The point of a schedule is not to control every single aspect of your day, but simply to not let your day control **you** so tightly. Time is your most precious asset, and you should think hard about what you choose to do with yours. Every so often you'll need to revisit your schedule and see where there is room for improvement, and weed out things that are not serving you.

Years ago, I used to be a major clean freak. My house had to be spotless and orderly, fresh and attractive. But then my son came along. That's when things changed. I had to make a choice. I had to ask, "Is being a clean freak serving me?" I found out it wasn't – it was taking time away from my family, and causing me guilt when I spent time scrubbing pots and pans instead of sitting down, hanging out with my son and husband. Being stressed, anxious, guilty, or angry about nothing specific – are all signs that something in your life is out of balance. When you begin feeling those things, consider setting aside a little time for yourself. As selfish as it may sound, you have to be sure that you are budgeting time for yourself, or you will have a bad attitude and no energy to take care of others – whether that is your job, your friendships, family, home or community. Perhaps "me" time for you is spending time with a girlfriend, going shopping or talking on the phone to your mom — it doesn't all have to be concentrated time spent in meditation or exercise. It is about relaxing, allowing yourself to become unburdened and really having the time to recharge.

What about when non-emergency situations come up — another mom calls and asks if you can drive the carpool instead, or your boss asks if you can stay late every night this week, and you just can't do it without serious help and rearranging of you life? Then it is time to have the courage to say "NO!" I understand, you are a woman, and by nature you are probably a pleaser — like me. But you truly cannot do it all. If you have afforded wiggle room in your schedule, maybe you can step up and drive the kids to soccer practice today, but if it is not going to work for you, you have to honor that and not try to conform to others' hopes and expectations. If something does present itself for your immediate attention, ask yourself the following questions to determine if you should do it, and when.

Does it have to be done right now?

Can I delegate this?

Can I fit this in later today?

Is this more important than the task I am currently doing?

You may want to consider delegating tasks to other people. I have just come through a very hectic and busy time in my life — authoring a book and launching a coaching program — it has been a whirlwind. I decided, before I began, on a date for all of my projects to be done, and then realized there was absolutely no way I could do all of it by myself, with any sort of quality in my work. So I asked for help. The people in my life: artists, web designers, marketing consultants, have been a godsend to me, and I must say that by delegating the things that I could afford to hire out, or that weren't my strongest suit, I was able to get more done in 2 months than I could have in an entire year!

So, how about you? Is there anything in your life you can delegate? Can your kids fold their own laundry? Is your husband willing to make dinner one night a week? Can you call another mom and see if she would take turns with you taking the kids to football practice? If you are a busy executive, a personal assistant to filter your emails, set up your appointments or run your errands will free you up to do what you are best at, and provide someone else with a livelihood. Don't be arrogant and think that "no one can do it as good as me." Maybe you are good at many things, but if you do TOO many things, you won't be excellent at any of them.

Don't be a passenger

You want to be in the driver's seat in your life, not sitting shotgun while it takes YOU for a ride. But to be in control of your life, you don't have to be a control freak. The first step to truly gaining the power to choose your own direction in life, is to realize that you have no control. I realized years ago when Brett died, that our control over life is at best tenuous, and at worst merely an illusion. Who among us hasn't experienced an unexpected loss, sudden illness, job layoff or financial hardship that seemingly came out of the blue? We have all been there, right? Sometimes, life totally blindsides you, and you are forced to face the reality that you really are not in charge of much of anything. The best way to gain control over the steering wheel is to admit the limits of your power to influence the ultimate course of events. Something else steers that – fate, God, the universe – whatever you want to call it. And it is up to you to surrender to that higher power in the world and let go of your need to manipulate and manage everything. You have to trust that everything will be okay – the money will come through, your heart will not permanently break, and that no matter what, at the end of any trial, life can be good, peaceful and okay. Your needs will be met, you will be whole and healthy. When I saw that picture of myself in the bathing suit all those years ago, I finally broke, and told God that I couldn't do it anymore. I'd tried everything and look where I was. I couldn't do it in my own power and strength, so I asked God to guide me, and help me fix this. Perhaps for you, it is your inner strength, your higher self that will get you through, and for others it may be trusting that the Universe wants harmony and balance. Whatever it may be – to be in control, you first have to realize that you have none.

Surrendering gives you freedom, and puts things in perspective. Clarity will come when you stop trying to control everything and you let your intuition lead you. And taking ownership for your faults, bad choices, behaviors and successes will allow you the grace to control the only thing you can – yourself. You never know what circumstances life will throw at you, but how you handle those circumstances is your choice. That is where the rubber meets the road: you in the driver's seat, choosing how to navigate life's obstacles. If someone comes at you in a negative or accusatory way, it is within your power to cool the fire or fan it. If you have made a mistake, it is within your power to become fearful and blame others, or to admit your wrongdoing and accept that you are imperfect and could have done better. When you are in conflict with co-workers, friends, family members or strangers and act in an honorable way towards them, you can diffuse a situation. I am not talking about being a peacekeeper, but a peacemaker. A peacekeeper is someone who will cover over or ignore monstrous problems and injustices, just to avoid a conflict. But a peacemaker sees their role in a situation and does their absolute best to be blameless within it. They may fight injustice, but it is done in a spirit of love and righteousness and not in anger or malice. Truly, your ability to control anyone or anything in your life is an illusion – the only thing you can direct is your own thoughts, feelings and behaviors.

DRIVING ON BUMPY ROADS

If life is going smoothly right now, hang on cause it's going to change. The only certainty in life is uncertainty. There are going to be bumps in the road, and major roadblocks that try to prevent you from traveling forward. Setbacks such as broken relationships, job loss, health issues – they're all there, and the fact is – God allows those things in your path because it is the only way you can get stronger. Believe it or not, things that seemingly get in your way in life, or bring you down, are actually blessings. The way to stay in the driver's seat of your own life is by choosing to see roadblocks as opportunities instead of hardships. For instance, if I had never been fat, or never had seen that photo of myself on the beach, it may have taken me much longer, and possibly never to surrender to the Universe and look inwardly for answers. My fat was a blessing. It helped me to change careers, to grow extensively on a personal level, to become more spiritual, to get closer to my husband, and much, much more. If I had been thin and "perfect" so to speak, I may never have done the work needed to create my own passionate and dynamic life!

What if life were perfect? You never argued, got sick, lost a job. You always had plenty of money and food and a nice place to live, all of your relationships were perfect, you felt loved and happy and safe.

What would be the impetus for you to evolve? How would you ever grow in patience? Where would you get the skills and empathy you need to comfort others experiencing hardship and pain? How would you gain wisdom on the things of this world? Not knowledge — wisdom, which only can come through age and experience?

There is a story I heard that illustrates this point. A man was walking in the woods one day and he spotted a chrysalis hanging from a low tree branch. He saw that it was wobbling to and fro, and realized that the butterfly inside was struggling to get out. Thinking that he could help, he took out his pocketknife and cut the chrysalis open. But the butterfly promptly fell to the ground and died. You see, the butterfly needs to struggle against the tough chrysalis shell, doing so floods his new wings with fluid that allows him to fly. Without the struggle, there is no transformation.

It is true for all of us, when you are driving down the road of life, there will be roadblocks. But what are you going to do about it? Turn around and drive home? Pout? NO! You are going to get out your map and find the way around the roadblock. Sometimes you'll be lucky, and a detour is marked for you, once in a while you may really have to study that map, and yet other times you will have to throw up your hands and look inside your intuition or ask your higher power to guide you. But you WILL get around it. Trust that. And believe that there is a point to it all — that through pain there will eventually be triumph. That without challenge, you will never grow. Think of what got you here — you were overweight and felt powerless. That was a major challenge in your life, but you read the map and navigated around the problem. And now you've come so far — becoming a healthier, stronger, and happier you, inside and out. You could not have had this life enriching experience on Interstate Vixen 12 if it weren't for that extra weight that you saw as a terrible burden.

THE GRATITUDE WHEEL
PART 3

In life, make it your goal to begin to think of roadblocks as opportunities instead of annoyances. Practice being grateful for the challenges you meet in life, at the time those challenges occur. It's okay to be let down, or sad or angry when things don't go as you'd planned or hoped. Having emotions, even the negative ones are part of our human nature. It is perfectly normal and okay to have those feelings. But when you do have those feelings of despair, take the time to just slow down and become aware... be in that moment and allow yourself a little time to process those feelings. Then, let it go and be grateful. What you don't want to do is hold onto those feelings of disappointment or sadness for long periods of time. Look for the beauty in what may seem at the moment to be ugly. It's not much different than when you did your mirroring exercises earlier in the program. Remember how, through daily practice, you eventually started seeing the beauty in yourself, rather than the flaws? The sooner you can let go of your hurt, anger or sadness and become grateful for those obstacles in life, the faster you will see the good and the opportunity in it. The more you practice this act of gratitude, the less time you will spend in a negative emotional space.

Be grateful for the opportunities life has presented you for growth. As my mother would say, "It gives you character". It isn't until you are hurting that you know the value of a good friend. It isn't until you are waiting for a blessing to come, that you learn the meaning of patience. It isn't until you don't know how you'll make it through tomorrow that you learn trust. Be grateful for life's irritations and major heart aches — they have all shaped who you are, and will continue to shape who you'll become.

Whenever you encounter a roadblock in your life, I want you to go to your journal or any piece of paper and write out what has happened. Just below it write: "I see this as an opportunity because..." and fill in the blank. Maybe you are too emotional and close to it to understand what the opportunity might be right now, that's okay — come back to it when you are able to think about the bigger picture. The more you practice this, the more it will become automatic. You'll be able to see the good, or at least hope for and expect the good that will come out of any situation. Maybe you lost your job, but how do you know a better one isn't coming? Maybe you fell off the wagon and gained 5 lbs, but now you realize that the commitment to yourself is worth it and you will continue caring for yourself in a healthy way for life. Even if you can't see it right now – good will come your way. Whether it is the patient endurance you will gain, the new perspective you'll see, or the better circumstance you'd have never dreamed of. Be grateful for difficulty, continue to cultivate an attitude of gratitude, and continue to look expectantly towards the future where there are new roads waiting to be explored.

You've been amazing! Celebrate this journey you've been on, and be grateful for your weight loss. Maybe you aren't there yet, but you are exactly where you are supposed to be right now. Be proud of these 12 weeks — you are healthier, fitter, and more mentally whole. You have left behind excess weight and emotional baggage, and obtained the skills you need to set more goals and achieve personal greatness. You have changed your inner woman as well as your outer one — you set a vision, followed the map and reached your first of many destinations on your lifelong journey of self-discovery and health. Are you perfect? No. Is this a perfect world? No. But, can you be happy? Yes! Do you love yourself? Yes! Are you going to continue what you started? Yes! You have reached Freedom, and now that you are free — go and share the journey with others. Show everyone in your life what a Vixen Unleashed looks like, and how they can become one too.

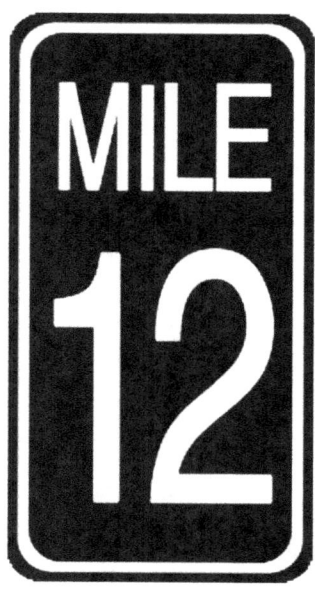

ACTION STEPS

- Create daily, weekly and monthly schedules that you can live with, budgeting plenty of time for the most important things – you and your loved ones
- Practice the 3rd component of the Gratitude Wheel, writing possible opportunities that will come from current hardships, in your journal. Continue to work parts 1 & 2 of the Gratitude Wheel and your mirroring exercises as well as your meditation.
- Continue to get 8-10 glasses of water per day, and eat healthy foods listed in the *High Octane Diet*.
- Continue to add to your exercise regime, mixing it up...and keeping at it.

Chapter 6

Freedom

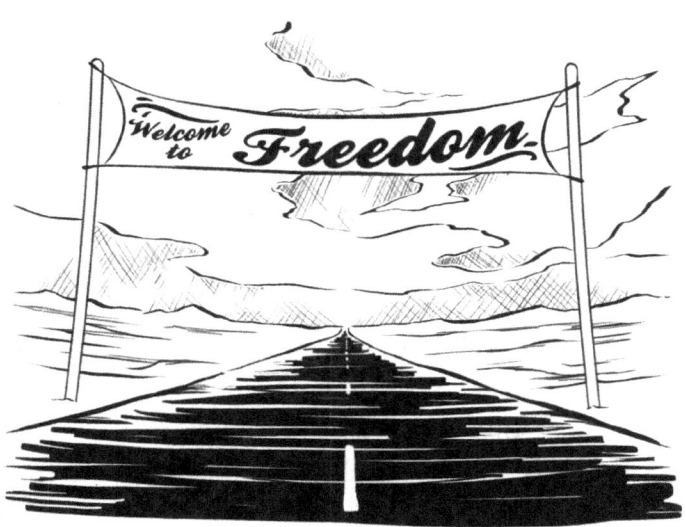

Throughout the past 12 weeks you have learned the importance of being grateful for what you do have, and for what you don't have just yet. You have learned how to nourish your body, mind and spirit. You have discovered who you really are, visualized your future self, set and achieved goals, and you've found strength, confidence and the "Vixen" within. You have implemented a program that includes a more balanced approach, using techniques that are both masculine and feminine in style. You have learned, yourself how to create a more synergistic and balanced lifestyle. Think about it… what changes have you been through? What "ah-ha" moments have you had? How do you feel about the woman you see in the mirror now, vs. the woman you saw 12 weeks ago? Whether or not you've reached your final or ultimate goal weight, if you've followed the map that I outlined for you, and have taken the time to implement your action steps at each Mile Marker, you have lost fat and made amazing progress in self-awareness, and have discovered some incredible things about yourself and your abilities. Just remember to continue to press forward using the tools and strategies that you learned along Interstate Vixen12. Remember that these tools can be used not only for weight loss, but also in every aspect of your life. Dream your vision. Set your goals. And as soon as you attain one goal, then begin creating even greater personal goals to strive for. But don't forget that your life journey is not just about setting and achieving goals. You can be a high achiever and still feel lost or stifled in life. By becoming introspective, being *honest* with yourself, knowing and consciously living by your core values, and following your instinct, you begin living a life filled with passion, purpose, and meaning. By listening to your Higher Power, and allowing that Divine Inner Spirit to guide you, rather than just beating yourself up because you're not "perfect" or because you're not "skinny", you will instinctively begin taking better care of yourself. Soon you'll find yourself following a more natural, peaceful path in life; you'll begin to see this in your relationships with people, with food, with your inner self and with your body. And the result of that will be a healthier, thinner, stronger BETTER version of YOU! By now, whether it is slightly, or immensely, my bet is that you are already seeing that better version of you. Even if you only took a few of the action steps, but still read through the entire book, you've learned a thing or two. You have taken one step closer to breaking the chains that bind you, and have begun unleashing your inner Vixen and experiencing Freedom. But it doesn't stop here. Change is a lifetime experience. It's inevitable. But to seek truth and self-awareness is a choice. Anyone can bury her head in the sand. It takes a brave woman to embrace change and *choose* to live life authentically. My BFF, Cindy once told me that I lead a very dynamic life. The definition of "dynamic" is constant change, activity or progress. When referenced to a person, it means to be full of energy and of positive attitude. As I was writing *Vixen Unleashed*, I kept asking myself, "If there is one thing that women can take away from reading this book, what is it?" Cindy's words kept popping back into my head, until one day it all became crystal clear. This book was created to help women lead dynamic lives, by giving them tools to discover their inner Vixen – that Divine Feminine within; and through the elements of nutrition, fitness and introspection, create a body that is reflective of their sexy, authentic self. I hope that from reading this book and following my program, you were able to do just that.

In the words of author, William S. Burroughs, "When you stop growing you start dying." So, keep growing, my friend...keep changing. Always strive to lead a passionate and dynamic life. And most importantly, be *sensual* in everything you do!

The End

"IQ" (INTROSPECTION QUIZ)

1. How long have you been overweight?

2. Is there a specific period of your life when you put on the majority of your weight? What was going on in your life at that time that may have contributed to your weight gain?

3. Name the top 3 stressors in your life right now. This could be anything: financial, relational, professional issues, or something else entirely. Once you have identified three sources of stress, think through why they are a source of anxiety and add those details.

4. Now take each of those 3 stressors and describe one way that you react as a result of that stress. (eg. If you explained that your finances are a problem for you because you've lost your job and are in debt, determine how you react when you write out your bills or fret over the future. Do you reach for the

ice cream after you've opened your checkbook? Do you lose sleep from worrying about retirement?)

5. Is there one area of your life where you really feel "stuck" or "trapped" , where you feel a dramatic shift needs to happen for you to be truly happy, that does NOT include losing weight or changing your body? Describe what that is and why.

6. Do you eat when you are bored, stressed, angry or happy?

7. If you answered "yes" to question 6, then you are eating for emotional reasons. Try to list at least 5 examples of times when you recognize that you binged or over-ate as the result of an emotion.

8. Describe in detail your eating habits. Describe what you eat, what time of day you eat your heaviest meals, your snack choices and what you eat to medicate your feelings.

9. To your knowledge, is there one particular thing that triggers you to overeat or consume unhealthy food? Be specific and give as much detail as possible.

10. What foods do you consider to be your "weakness" and your "go-to" comfort foods?

11. What are your favorite "healthy" foods?

12. Describe your current exercise habits – how often and what types including cardiovascular (such as aerobics or walking), weight bearing exercises (such as lifting weights or swimming) or mind-body exercises (such as yoga)?

13. How many times per week do you meditate? Have you ever meditated?

14. Taking in consideration your everyday work and home life, would you consider yourself sedentary, active, an athlete? Describe in detail your activity level.

15. On a scale from 1 – 10 (10 being that you love it and 1 being that you hate it) how do you like exercising?

16. If and when you exercise, when is your favorite time of day to exercise?

17. What is your most and least favorite form of exercise? (if none - please say so)

18. Name 3 things that you enjoy doing that involves movement, just for fun. (Example: dancing, hiking, cleaning house, dance video games, etc.)

19. Was there ever a time in your life when you feel that you were happy with your body size and your health? If so, describe that time in your life. What were you doing for a living? Where and with whom did you live? How old were you? If there was NEVER a time in your life when you were really happy with your body size and health, that's okay - many women have never been fully happy with their bodies.

20. Write down 5 typical "negative" things that you think or say about yourself and your body on a regular basis. For example: While grooming in the morning, you might say, "I hate my hair". Is that something that you find yourself doing often? Give 5 examples and the details.

21. Do you have any known food allergies or sensitivities?

22. Are you on any medications that could prevent you from eating a diet rich in protein, fruits and/or veggies?

23. Please list all foods that you absolutely do not like or do not eat.

24. Have you discussed with your doctor that you want to lose weight and are starting a new program?

25. When is the last time you had a complete blood-work analysis taken. What (if any) concerns did you or the doctor have as a result of that blood-work?

APPEARANCE

1. In detail, describe what your body looks like.

2. When you look in the mirror at your naked body, what physical traits do you NOT like?

3. When you look in the mirror at your naked body, what physical traits DO you like?

4. How many pounds (realistically) would you like to lose?

5. What size clothes would you (realistically) like to be in?

EMOTIONS

1. How does it make you feel when you look at yourself in the mirror?

2. Do you like how you look in clothes?

3. Have you ever felt ashamed or embarrassed by your appearance?

4. Describe the person that you see when you see yourself in photos?

5. On a scale of 1-10, how would you rate how you *feel* about what you LOOK like? (10 being that you feel great, 1 being you feel horrible)

6. On a scale from 1-10 (10 being the highest), how do you rate your desire to get thinner, stronger, and healthier?

CORE VALUES TEST

1. Name a time in the past when you felt your most beautiful, powerful and capable.

2. What accomplishment in life are you the most proud of? Why?

3. Who do you look up to the most? What characteristics does that person display?

4. Describe your best friend. What is it about them that you love?

5. Name five things that you absolutely hate (such as pollution, bullying, or material waste).

6. Is there anyone you dislike? What is it about them that puts you off?

7. Imagine you will die in 30 years, what is your legacy? What would you want to be remembered for?

8. Write a letter to your real or fictitious child to read as an adult. What advice would you share with them about life?

9. If you were suddenly rich and set for life, how would you use your time?

10. Create a fictitious place of safety in your mind – describe the location, who might you be with and how it makes you feel.

Try to be specific – if you are on a beach; describe the sand or the wind on your face.

11. Using the answers above, does anything stand out to you? Has a theme emerged? List any concepts or values that you see repeated.

From the following list, circle all the values that stand out to you, and add others as they occur to you. Don't over-think this. Just circle what jumps out at you. The best way to do this is to time yourself and complete the circling within 30 seconds.

Accomplishment	Freedom	Adventure	Money	Accountability
Kindness	Communication	Trust	Courage	Leadership
Spirituality	Peace	Bravery	Friendship	Benevolence
Relaxation	High rank	Morality	Risk Taking	Hard Work
Service	Efficiency	Organization	Recognition	Honesty
Discovery	Diversity	Intimacy	Invention	Tradition
Creativity	Excitement	Enjoyment	Justice	Sensuality
Knowledge	Wisdom	Motion	Duty	Education
Experience	Perfection	Possession	Health	Family
Logic	Energy	Practicality	Competition	Heroism
Control	Enthusiasm	Balance	Calm	Order
Cooperation	Punctuality	Strength	Perseverance	Maturity
Expression	Liberty	Radiance	Gratitude	Functioning
Giving	Focus	Devotion	Holiness	Brilliance
Elegance	Intuition	Security	Perceptiveness	Fidelity
Faith	Safety	Commitment	Love	Dignity
Fame	Beauty	Passion	Responsibility	Romance
Mastery	Affection	Poise	Influence	Confidence
Acceptance	Sharing	Voice	Self-worth	Independence

Working from the words you circled, list the ten values that stand out to you the most.

Now that we have looked into your potential future, your past and your present, use the answers from the first set of questions and the answers from the word exercise above to develop your list of 5 core values. You'll know it should make the list because you are repeatedly choosing the same ideas. Put them in descending order, beginning with the single value that is most important to you.

About the Author

As a young girl, Lynne Sadowski dreamed of being on stage. She had a passion for adventure and believed in the power of following dreams. This core philosophy landed Lynne in a career as an admissions representative at a private university, coaching and inspiring others to follow their passion. However, after 10 years of a sedentary lifestyle, Lynne found herself unhealthy, obese, and unhappy. She wasn't living an adventurous life, nor was she performing on stage. Then one day while taking a fitness class, Lynne looked into the mirror beyond her overweight body, and saw the vibrant and sexy woman she hadn't seen in many years. It was a pivotal moment, which led her to lose weight, get healthy, and start following her own dreams.

Today, Lynne Sadowski is co-owner of *Vixen Fitness*, an all women's fitness studio located in Orlando, Fl. She is also creator and founder of Lynne Sadowski's *Vixen Unleashed — Find it. Own it. Live it*. Her personal mission is to help women ignite their senses and lead passionate and dynamic lives in health, beauty, relationships, and career. She is living her passion of being on stage, speaking to audiences large and small, and she continues coaching people to help them live happier, healthier, and purpose-filled lives.

If you are ready to unleash your inner Vixen, and be a part of a coaching circle, home study course, or attend a *Vixen Unleashed* workshop or event in a city near you, go to: www.vixenunleashed.com to find out more!

Acknowledgments

First, before anything else, I'd like to thank Mom and Dad for believing in me and supporting my visions throughout my life. Thank you for being there for me in my darkest hours and in my brightest moments. I couldn't have asked for better parents. I'd also like to give the BIGGEST and most special thank you to my best friend, Cindy Baer. You are my rock, Cindy. Thank you for being there for me through everything and helping me stay focused on my vision. You are an amazing coach and incredible friend. And much gratitude, hugs, and love goes out to "The Circle" girls and Sedona Divas — Michelle, Lisa, Melissa, Kim, Sherri, Jennifer, Peggy, Theresa, Mildred, Mary, and Casey. And I'd like to express a BIG thank you to Michelle Phillips, author of *The Beauty Blueprint*, for your friendship and mentorship throughout the past year and a half. I'd like to give a VERY special thanks to my dear friend, Lisa Selow, author of *A Rebel Chick Mystic's Guide* for listening to me, guiding me and being so amazingly awesome. YOU ROCK, Lisa and I love you bunches! I'd also like to acknowledge contributor and wordsmith, Shelley Viggiano. Thank you, Shelley for helping me organize my thoughts, words, and writings, and for helping me put structure into my vision. You helped keep me moving steadily forward in this project, and I will be forever grateful. Of course, I'd like to give a big shout out, thank you, and LOTS of love to my family — my husband, Todd and my beautiful and amazing son, Jake, and the rest of the clan - Dave, Steve, my awesome sister, Carol, Marti, Alan, Candy, Alisa, Mike, Allison, Aleta, Albert, Buzz and Gerry. And thank you, Todd for being my photographer, my videographer, set-designer, cook, dishwasher, pool-boy, babysitter, pet-sitter, cleaning guy, handy man, breadwinner, and life partner. I love you from the bottom of my heart and thank God for you every day, and without you taking care of so much other "stuff" in my life, I wouldn't have been able to focus on this book! And then there is my rocker chick girlfriend, Carma! Thanks for always being there for me and believing in me! I would also like to extend immense gratitude for the girls who were there for me throughout many years and who were there for me like family in some of my toughest times…Sarah Webb, Tammy Nole, Debbie Hamilton, Minnie Lathe, and Kim Anderson. I also really want to thank Sherri Blye. You were by my side throughout the most challenging year in my life, which changed me spiritually. I honestly can't thank you enough for everything you've done for me. And thank you to my former co-workers at the university for inspiring me day after day, year after year and understood the power of following your dreams. I couldn't have worked with a more wonderful group of people and miss the times we spent together! Thank you Kitty, Sean, Shaun, Kevin, John, Holly, Aldania, Susan, Merigan, Lauren, Gianni, Carina, Patrick, Doug, Ben, Eric, Deborah, Debbie, Jack, Ryan and Jason. I'd also like to thank a few people who don't even know me, but who's teachings inspired me and my writings– Tony Robbins, Wayne Dyer, and of course, Marc David. Thank you to my newest friends and mentors, Tory Johnson from *Spark and Hustle* and *Good Morning America*, Cindy Morrison from *SocialVention*, and Coach Jenn Lee; what an amazing weekend together in New York, and I'm blessed to have you all in my life! Of course, I'd like to thank *Vixen Fitness* for those magical mirrors that helped me see the person I really am and continue empowering women daily! Thank you Allison Chapman for believing in me, supporting me and telling me about the gym that started it all. And thank you Jan and Vanessa, for our business partnership in *Vixen Fitness*. Thank you Courtney Sotack from Spa50 and Roxanne Gordon

(You GO! Rogographics -girl!) for creating the artwork on my book cover, and to Carol Hampshire for helping me put color and balance into my world. I want to give a HUGE thank you to Rae Edwards…a wonderful, talented, and beautiful Vixen who inspired me from day one. Thank you Rae, for the incredible illustrations you contributed to *Vixen Unleashed*, and for your patience and understanding throughout the whole thing. Finally, I'd like to thank all of the obstacles that came in the way of this project. Without them, I wouldn't have discovered the opportunities that allowed me to succeed far beyond my own imagination and dreams!

In Memory of Brett Geist

You are still missed by many; but your spirit
lives on, each and every day.

www.ingramcontent.com/pod-product-compliance
Lightning Source LLC
Chambersburg PA
CBHW070002200526
45794CB00001B/146